Pitfalls in Veterinary Surgery

Pitfalls in Veterinary Surgery

Edited by Geraldine B. Hunt

University of California at Davis
California, USA

WILEY Blackwell

This edition first published 2017
© 2017 John Wiley & Sons, Inc.

The right of Geraldine B. Hunt to be identified as the author of Pitfalls in Veterinary Surgery has been asserted in accordance with law.

Registered Office(s)
John Wiley & Sons, Inc., 111 River Street, Hoboken, NJ 07030, USA

Editorial Office
111 River Street, Hoboken, NJ 07030, USA
For details of our global editorial offices, customer services, and more information about Wiley products visit us at www.wiley.com.

Wiley also publishes its books in a variety of electronic formats and by print-on-demand. Some content that appears in standard print versions of this book may not be available in other formats.

Limit of Liability/Disclaimer of Warranty
The contents of this work are intended to further general scientific research, understanding, and discussion only and are not intended and should not be relied upon as recommending or promoting scientific method, diagnosis, or treatment by physicians for any particular patient. In view of ongoing research, equipment modifications, changes in governmental regulations, and the constant flow of information relating to the use of medicines, equipment, and devices, the reader is urged to review and evaluate the information provided in the package insert or instructions for each medicine, equipment, or device for, among other things, any changes in the instructions or indication of usage and for added warnings and precautions. While the publisher and authors have used their best efforts in preparing this work, they make no representations or warranties with respect to the accuracy or completeness of the contents of this work and specifically disclaim all warranties, including without limitation any implied warranties of merchantability or fitness for a particular purpose. No warranty may be created or extended by sales representatives, written sales materials or promotional statements for this work. The fact that an organization, website, or product is referred to in this work as a citation and/ or potential source of further information does not mean that the publisher and authors endorse the information or services the organization, website, or product may provide or recommendations it may make. This work is sold with the understanding that the publisher is not engaged in rendering professional services. The advice and strategies contained herein may not be suitable for your situation. You should consult with a specialist where appropriate. Further, readers should be aware that websites listed in this work may have changed or disappeared between when this work was written and when it is read. Neither the publisher nor authors shall be liable for any loss of profit or any other commercial damages, including but not limited to special, incidental, consequential, or other damages.

Library of Congress Cataloging-in-Publication data applied for

9781119241645 [Paperback]

Cover design: Wiley
Cover image: Courtesy of Geraldine B. Hunt

Set in 10/12pt Warnock by SPi Global, Pondicherry, India

Printed in Singapore by C.O.S. Printers Pte Ltd

10 9 8 7 6 5 4 3 2 1

Contents

Notes on Contributors

Geraldine B. Hunt

A child of Sydney's Northern Beaches, Geraldine Hunt graduated from the University of Sydney in 1983 and spent two years in small animal practice before commencing a PhD in cardiac electrophysiology, during which she learned about myocardial activation, open heart surgery, and critical care for thoracic patients. Following completion of the PhD, she worked for another year in small animal practice then moved on to a residency in small animal surgery. Having decided she wanted to become an academic, she took a position as lecturer in veterinary anatomy and, once she became a qualified Fellow of the Australian College of Veterinary Scientists, was also appointed as a visiting specialist to the University of Sydney Veterinary Teaching Hospital.

When a position as senior lecturer in small animal surgery became vacant, she moved full time to the Department of Veterinary Clinical Sciences. From there, she became head of small animal surgery and ultimately director of the Small Animal Teaching Hospital.

As a result of her early training in cardiac and vascular surgery, she developed a strong research interest in congenital cardiovascular diseases of dogs and cats. This developed into a particular focus on congenital portosystemic shunts. In 2008, deciding it was time to experience living and working in another country, she decided to make an even larger move, and left the University of Sydney to become Head of Small Animal Surgery at the University of California, Davis, USA.

Geraldine has been involved in training thousands of veterinary students and many surgical residents. Throughout all stages of her career, she has also maintained an interest in refining the discipline of surgery, and improving treatments for patients in private veterinary practice, and to this end has engaged in continuing education for veterinarians worldwide. This book is a continuation – and an extension – of those efforts.

Catherine F. Le Bars

Fascinated by the animal world from a very young age, Catherine Le Bars obtained her Bachelor of Veterinary Science from the University of Sydney in 1988. She spent her first four years working in mixed and companion animal practices, gaining experience and exposure to a varied client base and case load.

In 1992, she emigrated to the UK and traveled the country as a locum for two years, before settling into a busy Southampton practice. During her time there, she developed her skills in soft tissue surgery across a range of species, including companion animals, pocket pets, reptiles, and birds. Responsible for mentoring the veterinary graduates in the practice, Catherine was keen that they learned to walk before they ran, especially in the operating theater. This meant mastering the first principles of surgery and applying them to increasingly complicated procedures.

Catherine moved back to Australia in 2012 and established her own veterinary practice on the south coast of New South Wales. She takes pride in her role as a first opinion veterinary surgeon and always strives to achieve the best possible outcome for her patients and clients.

Julie M. Meadows

Julie Meadows graduated from the University of California School of Veterinary Medicine, Davis, in 1988. With great feeling for the human–animal bond she began general practice in California's Central Valley, where the clientele ranged from wealthy agricultural families and college professors to immigrant workers. At a time when specialty care was hours away and financial resources varied, she learned to appreciate the value of excellent communication with clients and a foundational understanding of her patients' medical problems in order to shepherd their health and that bond – what has now come to be called relationship-centered care.

Over 20 years in practice, including 10 years as a practice co-owner and two years teaching in a local veterinary technician program, she discovered the joy of sharing her values and experience with students and mentoring employees. With stars in her eyes for her alma mater, in 2008 she accepted a position as a clinical professor at UC Davis to develop its primary care program in response to a North American initiative to redirect veterinary education to entry level skills. There she and other pioneers shepherded the integration of core competencies such as communication and history-taking into the traditional curriculum across all four years of the program. She also built a robust general practice that allowed senior students to receive first presentation cases, including pediatrics and preventive healthcare, without house officers.

Julie returned to her professional roots in 2016, melding her loves of general practice and beaches by becoming lead veterinarian at a small practice in Cairns, Australia. Without the luxuries of having specialists in her building and access to advanced diagnostic capabilities, she has had to "practice what she preached" to students and is busy listening carefully to navigate international accents and new vocabulary. She spends her days with hands on her patients and exchanging knowledge with her new team as they work towards maintaining the human–animal bond in Australia.

Acknowledgments

To my parents, Susan and Michel, who always believed I could fly, and still feel I can soar higher. To my sister, Kate, my touchstone, and the best vet a coastal village could ever wish for. To my husband and partner in everything, George, who has helped me build a stable perch from which to spread my wings. To the many colleagues who supported me through the years, vets, techs, and others, who embraced me into the profession, taught me, challenged me, and boosted my spirits. To my students, the future of our profession, whose expressions of delight when they mastered the Ford interlocking suture made it all worthwhile. To my clients, who entrusted me with the lives of their dear companions. And to all my patients, who gave me so many opportunities to learn, improve, and teach, and who helped pave a smoother road for those to come. Names and some identifying details have been changed to protect patient confidentiality.

Preface

The thought struck me somewhere during the subcutaneous dissection.

I am a surgeon!

Not only a surgeon, but Faculty in one of the world's largest veterinary schools.

My patient was a skinny Rat Terrier called Rocket. Rocket hadn't moved quickly enough just over a week ago though, and found himself launched into low orbit by his neighbor's Prius.

He crash-landed on his stomach, which caused an ugly shearing injury to his groin; a ragged mouth exposing the fang-like shards of his shattered pubis.

Rocket was walking surprisingly well for a dog that had been so manhandled. His owners were maxed out on all their credit cards, so the emergency service opted for open wound management, which was complicated after only a few hours by a soaking flood of straw-colored fluid.

Somewhere in the mess that had once been Rocket's pubis, there was also a large hole in his urinary tract.

After reflecting on my career circumstances, my next thought was:

Why then, if I am such a well-credentialed surgeon, do I have so little idea of what to do next?

My student assistant – who had a keen interest in becoming a surgeon herself – watched intently as I dissected through a discolored mass of fat, edema, and hematoma. Our goal was to explore the caudal abdomen and see how much of Rocket's bladder and urethra was intact and then …

And then what, exactly?

This was truly exploratory. There had been no money for advanced imaging, so I really didn't know what I was going to find. And it was purely a salvage procedure; the owners could not afford stents or bypass conduits, or delicate reconstructive surgery which might or might not work. Rocket's options were very restricted.

Later, after I had located the transected end of the urethra just caudal to the prostate, brought it through the ventral abdominal wall, and anastomosed it to the caudal fornix of Rocket's prepuce[1] (Figure P.1), the student said, "Wow! I have never seen that before!"

"Neither have I."

She grinned. "Yeah, right."

"No, I'm serious."

She stared at me, mouth slightly open, "But you just … you went ahead and did it, as if you'd done it a hundred times before. How do you know what to do?"

It was a good question. How *did* I know what to do, and how to do it? It was not as simple as opening a book and following the instructions. In reality, it was a synthesis of my experiences – good and bad – with many patients. Putting my textbook knowledge into a practical context to solve a new problem.

1 Bradley RL. Prepubic urethrostomy: an acceptable urinary diversion technique. *Problems in Veterinary Medicine* 1989; 1: 120–127.

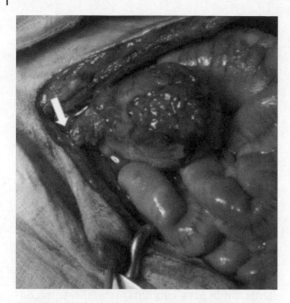

Figure P.1 Prepubic anastomosis of the prostatic urethra to the prepuce (arrow) in a dog following trauma.

I eventually answered, "I have some tricks I learned through the years."

"Can you teach me?"

Another good question. It took three more years and some careful thinking to answer it, but here goes …

1

"Can't You Do Anything Right?"

The Shocking Realization That I Was Not Perfect

My father likes to introduce me as the vet who put the parrot's leg on backwards.

Having invested so much emotional and financial capital in my education, I am perplexed that my parents should find amusement in this embarrassing moment of my budding veterinary career. Surely they should inform their friends of my years of training, or all the letters following my name, or my position as a professor of surgery. But I am doomed to being defined in my family's eyes by one small yet highly visible complication (I think there were extenuating circumstances, but you can make up your own mind later).

Having evolved from a childhood dream of palaeontology (which lost its appeal once I realized dinosaurs and humans never cohabited the planet), I cycled through visions of African exploration to becoming a marine scientist, a forensic pathologist and – finally – a jet-setting equine veterinarian (Figure 1.1). Veterinary science would suit me, I decided. I preferred animals to people: people were too focused on themselves, they held silly ideas and misconceptions, and they complained too much. Ironic then, that the first harsh criticism of my career came directly from one of my animal patients.

Mrs. Sofel was a long-term client of the small animal practice that employed me immediately after graduation. She was probably only in her mid-sixties but looked about a hundred to a young veterinarian fresh out of university. Our relationship did not get off to a particularly good start, as she took one look at me when I entered the consulting room and wanted to know what I had "done with Dr. Davidson."

"Dr. Davidson is on holiday for 2 weeks," I replied.

"Well, I suppose you'll just have to do, then," she sniffed. She usually came in trailing a Cushingoid Maltese with more warts than teeth, but this time she swung a large birdcage onto the examination table. I realized her frail appearance belied great strength; a conclusion that did little to sooth my new-graduate nerves. The birdcage contained a huge, sulphur-crested cockatoo.

"Oscar has a lump," said Mrs. Sofel.

For a moment, I was speechless; not because Oscar was a bird, or because his beak resembled a large pair of garden shears, but because he was almost completely bald. I quickly diagnosed him as suffering from beak and feather disease. Actually, it was just about the only disease I could remember from my avian medicine lectures at that particular moment. I stared at Oscar, who stared back; his beady black eye encircled by leathery grey skin. He looked little like a bird, and much more like some form of mutant dinosaur. The effect was complete when he raised the lone yellow feather on the crest of his head, and screeched. I practically hit the ceiling.

"It needs to be removed," Mrs. Sofel announced.

My heart already pounding, I was further horrified to realize she was talking not about the single head feather which had so captured my attention, but about a large, egg-shaped mass protruding from Oscar's rump.

Pitfalls in Veterinary Surgery, First Edition. Edited by Geraldine B. Hunt.
© 2017 John Wiley & Sons, Inc. Published 2017 by John Wiley & Sons, Inc.

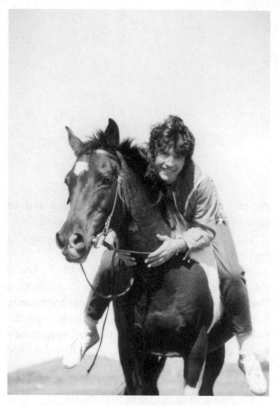

Figure 1.1 A young "Dr. Hunt," quite obviously destined to become a small animal surgeon.

My main comfort at this point was that I had so little experience I did not yet know what to be frightened of. I knew how to anesthetize birds: we had knocked out chickens in a practical class at uni and successfully woken most of them up again. And I'd had a good training in basic surgery, so I had a rough idea of how to remove lumps. I wasn't quite sure how I was going to get Oscar out the cage in order to do either of the above, but I was sure I could cross that hurdle when I came to it.

"Well, um, yes ... we can do that," I said.

"When and how much?" These were the days before computerized medical records, appointment systems, or account-keeping programs, so I made a quick escape to the reception desk to find the answers. Thank goodness for Theresa, our wonderful receptionist and long-term backbone of the practice. She gave me the information I needed (I suspect she would also have been able to tell me what drugs and surgical instruments to use, had I only asked).

Mrs. Sofel and I agreed on a price, and a date when Dr. Davidson was back in clinic, and she swept Oscar's cage up and turned on her heel. But Oscar was not finished. He craned his neck to look back at me, and the crest feather slowly elevated again. I braced myself for the parting screech, but instead Oscar said in his parrot's voice (closely resembling that of an old woman), *"Can't you do anything right?"*

I stared at Mrs. Sofel, who said nothing. I had the uncanny sense that Oscar and his owner had formed a telepathic bond. Mrs. Sofel sniffed again and sailed from the waiting room, leaving me struggling for words. I suspect that particular phrase was heard frequently by those in her company, and never received a satisfactory answer.

Whatever the explanation, Oscar's question proved sadly prophetic when we masked him down two weeks later, and he promptly died. In retrospect, we should have asked Theresa to do it. She later told me that parrots "always died" when anesthetized and left me wondering how many times Dr. Davidson had proven that particular theory.

Needless to say, Mrs. Sofel blamed me for Oscar's death simply by virtue of my proximity to the saintly Dr. Davidson on the fateful day, and refused to allow me near any of her *"other* pets *ever* again." Although such banishment was a blow to my ego, it was not an entirely unwelcome outcome, all things considered.

After incubation in primary school, hatching from high school, and being "fledged" at university, I had spent 18 years in the educational nest, so to speak. Surely that rendered me capable of doing a lot of things "right," contrary to Oscar's observation? Having finally launched into my career with the tenuous belief I would become airborne, I quickly realized I had not flown from the nest so much as staggered out of it, and been fortunate enough to bounce when I hit the ground.

I am sure I was a great success at many things in my early days as a veterinarian. But for some reason the comfort of our successes fades quickly, while our failures remain to irritate us, as surely as Oscar's diseased feathers had irritated him. At least Oscar was able to pull his feathers out. Looking back on all those mystery patients, unfathomable clients, the questions for which the textbooks provided no answer, all those mistakes I made, and all the things I had to learn the hard way, I do wonder how different my years of practice might have been if I had the knowledge then that I have now.

If only I had known!

We acquire knowledge in many different ways. We have different learning styles. We memorize things by rote, but we truly learn them when we have the chance to apply them. Our profession is a fluid mix of thinking and "doing"; very much dependent on the type of case and its unique circumstances. Some patients fit the textbook description perfectly, whereas others break all the rules. Clients have particular needs and restrictions when managing their pets, and there is always the issue of finance. Sometimes, I suspected the tides or phase of the moon dictated whether things went according to plan. Were the stars aligned? Did I wear my lucky socks to work that morning? Faced with such a complex system, there is only so much our university professors and textbooks can teach us.

Our successes involve a large portion of "seat of our pants" intuition and good luck. Scientific and evidence-based as our profession has become, we will always have to learn some things by trial and error, by simply seeing what works and what does not. Textbooks give us a definitive description, a clear way to proceed with diagnosis and treatment, and a neat explanation for cause and effect. We try to make cases fit the textbook description, or vice versa, and mentally file away inconvenient pieces of information that don't fit in the hope that the abnormalities will either go away on their own or make sense once the patient gets better, or maybe when we've got more experience. What textbooks usually don't show us, though, is the process their authors went through to evolve

the crisp conclusions they share in print. They tell us about the sum total of their experience, and tend not to dwell on the cases that broke the rules.

Speaking to a group of general practitioners in rural Australia some years ago, I shared the story of a truly perplexing case. This case had no fairy tale ending, we made many mis-steps along the way, and the ultimate answer was only revealed in the postmortem room. Standing beside me in the lunchtime coffee line, one of the older vets said:

"I liked your lecture. It gave me a lot of hope."
"That's good to hear. And why was that?"
"I realized you specialists don't have all the answers, either."

I have heard this many times since; from students, junior academics and vets in practice. There is an impression that after a certain level of training, when you achieve fellowship or diplomate status, somehow you know all there is to know, and you never screw up.

It is comforting to the people reading the textbooks, and listening to the lectures, that they aren't the only ones who scratch their heads, find test results that defy explanation, draw the wrong conclusion, agonize over their treatment plan, or struggle for ideas when their plans don't work.

When I ask my colleagues in specialty practice whether they have made mistakes, most of them are quick to say, "Hell, yes!" or "My oath!" (depending on which side of the Pacific they come from). But that is not always the impression we give when we deliver our lectures or write our textbook chapters. We talk about our successes, show the best photographs, sanitize our complications, and generally present a stylized version of what can be a slow, frustrating, confusing, and sometimes downright messy process.

Unpalatable as it is to admit, our cases don't always go well. Most of us are happy to learn from someone else's mistakes, but it is particularly intimidating to confront your own mistakes honestly. Gruelling as it can be, through my years as an academic and a teacher of veterinarians, I have reaped an ironic reward from sharing my low moments with others and thus allowing them to learn.

Of course, being a veterinarian is not just about the animals. In a perfect world, desperate clients would bring an ailing pet to us and take a healthy one home again after showering us with gratitude and admiration, and full payment of their bill. Reality, however, is not quite so Disneyesque. My experience with Mrs. Sofel was more than simply a lesson in how easily I could fall foul of others. In Mrs. Sofel, I had my first encounter with the client whose sole aim seemed to be to make my life miserable. These clients rarely had a kind word to say, and were capable of finding fault in the most benign of circumstances (Oscar's death aside, which was understandably devastating for everyone). I wondered what it was about me that caused some people to be so very difficult, and I wanted so very badly to defend myself. Couldn't they see that I was trying my best to help them and their pets? Where was the gratitude? The admiration? How dare they tell me how to treat their pet after I spent five years in veterinary school?

I stormed into the treatment room one day after being lectured on how to clip a Yorkshire Terrier's nails.

"Looks like that appointment went well," my nurse, Karen, commented wryly as I hurled the nail scissors into the sink.

"That woman is such a ...," I bit my lip. My suspicions about the human race were being confirmed, but my plan of avoiding interpersonal conflict by becoming a veterinarian was rapidly unraveling. "What did I do to deserve that?"

Karen said nothing, merely tapped a photocopied page stuck to the wall above the telephone. It was titled, "Why It Is Not About You." One of the practice partners posted it after attending a management course. The gist was that when people become aggressive, it is more often about their personality, or what is happening in their lives, than a personal attack on you.

It recommended taking time out to think about things from the other person's perspective, and suggested some explanations:

1) In pain
2) Fearful
3) Stressed
4) Grieving
5) Financial trouble
6) Mental illness.

When we had a difficult interaction, we would take refuge in the back room and try to work out which explanation might best fit that person. It was a great way to defuse the angst, refocus ourselves on the patient and what it needed, and alleviate the often overwhelming desire to march back out and tell our clients why they were being so totally unfair. In the years before "doctoring" and "client management" courses in vet school, these client hostilities took me by complete surprise, and this simple printout was my first introduction to the complex and fascinating science of human behavior.

Naturally, we had some clients who did not seem to fit any of the categories on the printout, and thus someone had penciled at the bottom:

7) Just plain mean
8) Absolute nutter.

As time went on, I discovered that this was only one small piece of a far more complex puzzle, and as my career took me deeper into the specialty of small animal surgery, with its milieu of emotion-charged circumstances and highly invested clients, I would face gradually escalating surgical challenges, accompanied by rich opportunities for honing my people skills.

In the following chapters I share my experiences about the "pitfalls" of small animal surgery: the things I learned the hard way, the cases that still haunt me, the clients I worked hard to "unpuzzle," and some bright successes when things went exceptionally well. And mine is not an experience confined to the ivory towers of the university, as you will hear from others who have contributed their own stories and insights to this book.

2

Beastly Bellies

Sunday nights were some of our busiest at the regional practice in which I worked for my first two years. We were the only show in town for after-hours coverage once everyone else knocked off for the weekend and switched their phones to the answering machine.

There were many dog fanciers around the Canberra area, and during show season the required chemistry often failed to develop during a romantic weekend and the stud male did not breed the visiting bitch. This prompted a frantic call for emergency insemination before the bitch was driven home again. I had a rough idea of how to collect semen and perform artificial insemination, so Sunday night often found me crouched beneath a perplexed Maltese or Weimaraner dog, feverishly trying to press the right buttons. A quick glance at the resultant sample under the microscope to check for motility, and the accompanying bitch was inseminated by means of a syringe and urinary catheter. Amazingly, some of these emergency "matings" resulted in live puppies.

The unforseen consequence of these reproductive rescues was that our practice became known as the "go to" place for artificial insemination, and we started attracting non-emergency cases.

Mr. Fortescue, from Brindabella Kennels, brought his Bichon Frise couple to us because he didn't like to see them "doing that nasty stuff." Mrs. Grande marched in her German Shepherd, Pinetree Macho III, for semen collection because he just wasn't interested in her stud bitches.

We stumbled fortuitously on a solution for Macho's ennui the day we had Fortescue and Grande dogs in the practice at the same time and Macho concluded that Brindabella Perfect Muffin was his ideal Playboy centerfold. We scrambled to prevent some spontaneous "nastiness" from occurring in the middle of the treatment room, but it made our job of collecting from the German Shepherd a whole lot easier. Each time Macho came in for semen collection from then on, we endeavored to produce a small white fluffy "teaser," and it never failed to get his juices flowing. Despite being occasionally fruitful, and spawning ageless practice jokes, these cases did not impregnate me with the desire to become a theriogenologist, hence you are not reading memoirs of my career in reproduction. They did, however, teach me that sometimes you just have to give things a shot and you will occasionally surprise yourself.

An owner recently said one of the things he really appreciated about his vet was that they were at least prepared to "try." The trick is to know your limitations, and have a good feeling for the potential consequences. For the great proportion of pets whose owners will never be able to spend the time or money on referral to a specialist center, this is equally important whether you are a boarded surgeon or a general veterinarian in a one-person rural mixed practice. Working out which cases you should keep in your practice, which ones you should refer, and which cases are appropriate for surgery at all takes experience and self-reflection, as you will see in the following chapters.

Pitfalls in Veterinary Surgery, First Edition. Edited by Geraldine B. Hunt.
© 2017 John Wiley & Sons, Inc. Published 2017 by John Wiley & Sons, Inc.

One particular Sunday night during my first year in practice sticks with me for many reasons. The weather was foul: winters in Canberra were cold and often wet. We rarely got the snow that blanketed the nearby Australian "Alps" but, having swept across the high country, the freezing winds and turgid clouds spent themselves over Australia's capital city. On this night, it was blowing a gale and a mixture of rain and sleet beat against the windows. We had a ward full of dogs and nowhere to dry the washing, so we hung it across the treatment room on a spider's web of ropes strung between cages. The combination of a fan-forced heater and damp washing filled the room with a humid, musty fug that made it seem less like a veterinary practice and more like some inner-city sweat shop.

We had just finished stabilizing a Border Collie with metaldehyde poisoning, who had covered much of the floor, one wall, and my trousers in a black–green slime as he purged snail bait and activated charcoal from both ends. The renal failure cat was crouched in the back of its cage; unkempt coat sticking up like porcupine quills, but not as spiky as we found his teeth and claws to be as we fiddled with his intravenous catheter to keep the fluids dripping. I was savoring a brief respite and looking forward to dressing the scratch marks on my arms and changing into clean clothes when the doorbell rang.

My newest patient was a 10-and-a-half-year-old black Labrador who'd chosen that afternoon to go down acutely. His middle-aged owner carried him in; no small feat, as this dog was clearly a prodigious eater. The labored breathing, pale gums, and thready pulse suggested Bill was really struggling, and Roger – the dog – didn't look much better. I encouraged Bill to lay Roger on the waiting room floor, before we ended up with two emergency cases on our hands.

As Roger lay flat out beside the fish tank, his abdomen was grossly distended, even accounting for his body condition score of 11. It was firm and tight, and Roger groaned when I palpated it.

"Acute abdomen," I said, envisioning necrotizing pancreatitis or septic peritonitis.

"He's been getting quieter for a few days," said Bill, who had now caught his breath and looked less like he was about to suffer an acute event of his own. "And he's been straining a lot."

I added urethral obstruction to my list of differentials.

"And his gums have been pale."

Bleeding splenic hemangioscaroma, surely!

"We've had him on a diet. We thought his weight was getting the better of him. Then his tummy suddenly swelled up."

I settled on a diagnosis of gastric dilatation volvulus (GDV), and was running through a mental checklist in preparation for anesthesia and surgery, but wanted to make sure Roger's stomach actually was full of gas before I stuck a needle in. We had no ultrasound machine in those early days, so our in-house diagnostics were limited to a radiograph and some very basic blood work. We rolled Roger onto a stretcher and took him through to the X-ray room. I snapped a lateral radiograph and left Bill with his recumbent mate while I locked myself in the dark cave. When I emerged 10 or so minutes later, imbued with the vinegar-reek of developing fluid, I held the still-damp radiograph to the light. I saw neither the radiolucent double-bubble of GDV, nor the ground-glass appearance of hemoabdomen. Rather, Roger's abdomen seemed full of something resembling aggregate pavement.

"What's he been eating?"

"You mean, what *hasn't* he been eating?" Bill shook his head. "He got into the pantry yesterday afternoon. Made a shocking mess."

Gastrointestinal foreign body! I started towards the autoclave, then hesitated. I had hoped my first exploratory laparotomy might occur during the day, and in the presence of a more experienced colleague. Was I about to make the right decision? It seemed clear that Roger was full of something that needed to be removed, but was surgery the answer?

I belatedly decided to finish my physical examination, and pulled on a glove to do a rectal exam.

The cause of Roger's distress soon became evident; my finger emerged encased in a clay-like material liberally reinforced with vegetable husks. On further interrogation regarding the "shocking mess" in Bill's pantry, it became evident Roger was suffering an emergency case of constipation arising from his misguided notion that a starving dog might save its life by devouring two kilograms of pumpkin seeds.

Shifting the offending vegetation took most of the evening, a large amount of warm soapy water, contributed greatly to the Border Collie's efforts in resurfacing the floor, and added at least one string of wet towels to our attempt at creating an indoor rainforest. I hoped to see orchids sprouting from the walls at any time, but eventually had to settle for a patchy layer of mold.

It was worth it though, when Roger trotted out the door the next morning, albeit with a sheepish expression and a phobia about anyone approaching his back end. The abdominal distention was only minimally reduced, and we suggested the owners continue the diet and bulk it out with mashed pumpkin so Roger did not feel compelled to fill the empty hole in his belly with anything that came within range of his mouth.

Roger was my first lesson in the value of rectal examination. We are taught that it is integral to the physical examination, but how often do we actually perform it thoroughly? The dog's too wriggly, we have four clients in the waiting room, and the owner is focused on the lump on the head.

In vet school, my clinic team examined a Dalmation presented for anxiety and panting. When history and physical examination did not yield a definitive diagnosis, we auscultated the chest, checked the cranial nerves, drew blood for hematology and biochemistry, and went away to await the results, leaving one of our fellow students to babysit the dog in the treatment room. Ten minutes later, a student from another team flew in: "You have to see this!"

We raced back in time to watch John deliver a foul-smelling object from the dog's anus. For want of anything else to do, he had decided to perform a rectal exam, and been rewarded with the tail end of a length of fabric. As nobody had ever told us about intestinal plication or perforation resulting from linear foreign bodies, the most natural thing seemed to be to pull it out. We watched John pull and pull, like a magician drawing a scarf from a hat, until he relieved the dog of a complete pair of panty hose. Needless to say, he was the hero of the hour, and of course we did not know how close he had come to creating a rectal prolapse, or maybe even an ileocolic intussusception.

Suffering from dizzy spells as a first year PhD student, I went to my local general practitioner for a checkup. After taking my blood pressure and looking in my ears, he pulled on an exam glove. I wasn't sure which particular cause of vertigo he was searching for in that manner, but he said, "If you don't put your finger in it, you'll put your foot in it."

I can't say I appreciated this GP's overly thorough investigation of my vestibular system, especially when he terminated the short consultation by advising me to cut back on coffee, but it did highlight the role of rectal examination in a thorough work up and also taught me the benefit of clearly explaining the rationale for your various investigations to the subject (or in our case, its owner).

While most rectal examinations do not yield such a rewarding outcome as John's Dalmation, or Roger the pantry raider, I can remember a handful of patients where it was not only the key part of the diagnosis, but failing to do it led to serious delays in diagnosis and treatment: they included a Labrador treated medically for recurrent constipation caused by a pelvic lipoma, a Cocker Spaniel with polyuria and polydipsia caused by an anal sac adenocarcinoma, and a Kelpie cross evaluated for syncope during defecation, whose advanced rectal adenocarcinoma was not identified until after her pacemaker was implanted.

In the week following Roger's de-obstruction, I saw Barney, another 10-year-old Labrador, with an almost identical presentation: gaining weight and becoming more and more lethargic, despite being on a diet for the last four weeks. His abdomen was distended, but this time the radiograph showed a soft tissue mass and we diagnosed a splenic tumor. This time we really were headed into the operating theater.

I had spayed a couple of cats and dogs, but wasn't that familiar with surgery of the abdomen, but I thought I should be able to find the spleen, and I knew how to tie ligatures, so how hard could it be? We anesthetized and prepped Barney and I performed a textbook ventral midline incision into the abdomen. You might have experienced the "detour" signs that direct you down a poorly lit secondary road and then vanish, leaving you lost in the dark; well, that's about where any resemblance to what I had seen in a textbook ceased. I'm not sure what I expected, but I suspect it was something looking vaguely like the spleen from Miller's *Anatomy of the Dog*, with color-marked hilar vessels and neatly defined gastrosplenic attachments. What emerged from Barney's abdomen proved to be a lobulated monster liberally covered with rope-like veins and arteries, and smothered in discolored omentum. I stared at it, waiting for inspiration.

None was forthcoming from elsewhere, so I had to work it out on my own.

I'll explore the abdomen, I thought, *and see what it's attached to.*

I could not even slide my hands around the mass, despite the fact that I had incised from xiphoid to umbilicus.

Extend the incision caudally, I thought, and promptly cut the preputial artery and vein. The exercise of clamping and ligating those vessels bought me more time to think, and sweat. It was my first taste of that dry-mouthed, hollow feeling when you realize you don't actually know what to do next.

Extending the incision didn't improve my visualization very much as everything seemed attached to everything else (Figure 2.1). My next bright idea was to lift the mass out of the abdomen. It would not budge. The attempt merely served to rupture one of the fragile veins

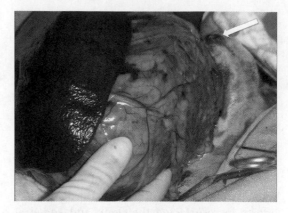

Figure 2.1 The trick with massive splenic tumours is to make a long enough incision. This incision extends well past the prepuce (arrow), yet it is still difficult to exteriorize this tumor.

snaking across its capsule, earning me some more perspiration time as I got the bleeding under control.

Realizing that there was no easy way to do this, I decided to simply start ligating blood vessels, and hope that eventually I would get around the thing. Two and a half hours and about three meters of surgical gut later, I finally hefted the massive splenic tumor out of the dog and was hugely relieved when the rest of the abdominal contents remained where they were supposed to be.

Barney was tachycardic, which we addressed with large amounts of PlasmaLyte, but he was alive and recovered slowly from anesthesia and we patted ourselves on the back. The next morning, Barney was stretched out in his cage with ghost-white mucous membranes. I sacrificed a goodly portion of his few remaining red blood cells in order to show that he had an hematocrit of 6%. As blood transfusions were beyond the scope of our practice, we gave him an iron tablet and hoped for the best. The fact that he was too anemic to stand fortunately did not prevent this Labrador from wolfing down a couple of kangaroo steaks. Removing the massive tumor from his abdomen restored his trim waistline, and earned him a pardon from his rigid diet of the last few weeks. We discharged him – weak but happy – a couple of days later and I had learned another major lesson: when you don't know what to do next, sometimes you just have to start somewhere and make slow and steady progress until you get where you need to be.

We encounter many large abdominal masses in dogs and cats. Fortunately, most of them are splenic in origin, mobile, and lift fairly easily from the abdomen, their stretched pedicle presenting itself neatly for ligation. But abdominal masses are not all like that, and developing a strategy for tackling the less convenient ones can make it less stressful and more effective.

Here are a couple of questions to ask yourself when deciding on your strategy.

1) *Is my incision going to give me satisfactory access?* The traditional stem-to-stern ventral midline incision will serve for many mid-abdominal masses, but does not work well for large lateral liver or kidney masses. You can join a ventral midline incision with a paracostal incision, creating a flap of lateral abdominal wall and greatly improving access to the left or right craniodorsal abdomen. But only if you clip the patient high enough laterally on each side before draping it!
2) *Is the mass solid or cavitated?* My main concern is how richly a mass is supplied with blood vessels. It can be difficult to determine whether the great vessels of the abdomen actually run through a large mass, or are innocent bystanders. Contrast-enhanced computed tomography (CT) has become a mainstay of evaluation for abdominal masses in people and animals. Many times we will send a patient for a CT to "work out whether the mass is resectable or not." CT is invaluable for evaluating the vascularity of a tumor, and its relationship to the great vessels, but it does not necessarily help determine whether it is adherent to the surrounding structures, and how easily they might be separated.

I tell my owners that I use CT to decide whether a mass is *not* resectable (i.e., are critical structures intimately associated with it, precluding its removal without unacceptable morbidity?) but my test of choice about whether something can really be removed is to physically put my hands around the mass and see whether I can lift it out of the abdomen.

The moral of all this? Do not give up until you have either proven that the mass cannot be separated from other vital structures or that it will not lift out of the abdomen, allowing the normal structures to remain in situ and demonstrating the attachments that need to be ligated (Figure 2.2). Sometimes your patients will surprise you.

(A)

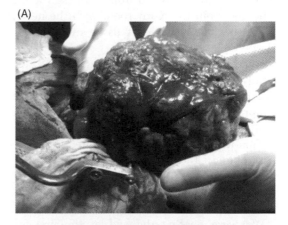

(B)

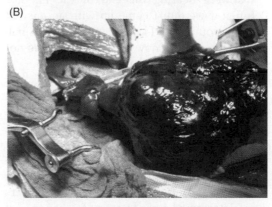

Figure 2.2 (A) Sometimes the "resectability" of a mass can only be assessed by sliding your fingers around it and lifting it out. (B) This liver mass was easily exteriorized, revealing a narrow pedicle that could be clamped and ligated.

At 16 years of age, Petunia was a venerable old lady as cats go when she was presented for evaluation of her "expanding waistline." This was an understatement, as Petunia resembled a butternut squash. She was the same color too, suggesting that whatever had taken up residence in her abdomen was engaged in an intimate relationship with her common bile duct. Radiographs were not helpful. At her age, Petunia had developed a strong opinion of what she should and should not be required to endure, and lying on her side was one of the latter. After struggling for some time, and spending a hundred odd dollars of the owner's money to achieve a radiograph resembling one of those torticollic dinosaur fossils chiseled from Chinese rock, I emerged from the X-ray room with the news, "Yes, she has a large soft tissue mass in her abdomen."

Her owners were gracious enough to nod solemnly in response to this confirmation that Petunia's advanced state of turgidity was indeed abnormal. They also shared the information that, "The other vet said the same thing."

This was a strong clue that mine wasn't the first opinion they had sought, and they confirmed this with, "They said it was too advanced for them to operate, but we've come to the university to make sure."

We were nearing the end of the line for Petunia; if we didn't come up with an answer, nobody would. And I knew enough about small animal practice by now to realize this was not going to be a simple splenic tumor.

Fortunately, the University of Sydney had excellent ultrasonographers, who confirmed that the mass occupying the vast majority of Petunia's peritoneal cavity was filled with fluid. CT was a glimmer on the horizon, but not yet a reality for our practice, so three-dimensional imaging was out of the question. But Petunia was running out of options, and her owners were determined to at least try to diagnose, if not resolve, her problem, so we scheduled her for surgery. I had not yet formulated any particular strategy for approaching the non-standard abdominal mass, so started with the basic ventral midline incision. We positioned Petunia obliquely on the table in the hope that whatever blood was squeezing through her caudal vena cava should not be further challenged by the dead weight of her alien passenger (Figure 2.3A).

Petunia's body wall was stretched enough to be semitranslucent, and parted almost gratefully beneath my scalpel to extrude a glistening gray dome (Figure 2.3B). At the caudal-most extent of the incision, a tangle of unnaturally flattened jejunum made its bid for freedom, and Petunia's blood pressure shot up momentarily as blood began to return from the caudal half of her body. With the rock-hard object now half in and half out of the peritoneal cavity, I had the faintly hysterical vision of walking out to reception to report to the waiting owners that, "Yes, I am now convinced. Petunia has a large soft tissue mass in her abdomen!"

The mass was solid and sessile, and would not shift one way or the other. For some strange

(A)

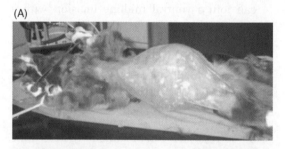

(B)

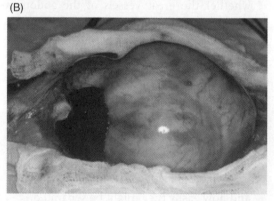

Figure 2.3 (A) Grossly distended abdomen in a cat with a biliary cyst. (B) Appearance of the cyst upon opening the abdomen.

reason that I still don't understand, we had not seen fit to aspirate it during the ultrasound examination, and I had no idea what sort of fluid it actually contained, although I was working on the presumption that it was bile, and this was some form of extravagant biliary cystadenoma. Did I think I really had a chance of removing it? In retrospect, I don't think so, but we were not prepared to give up on Petunia unless we knew for sure.

Having seen my adversary in the flesh – so to speak – I began to think that perhaps we'd gone as far as we could go. I had no idea what this thing was growing from, or how invasive it was. I had no idea what other structures I might have to sacrifice in order to remove it. If only it were a little smaller, so I could look around the sides and see what was happening in the abdomen. In a fortuitous coalition of random thoughts, I decided to aspirate the cyst to confirm the fluid as bile and as I was preparing to do this, I thought, *If it is bile, why not drain it completely and see whether that helps me explore the abdomen?*

This might seem self-evident, but when you are confronted with the unexpected in surgery you don't always think clearly. In many cases, I only worked out the ideal strategy in retrospect.

To my great surprise, when I plunged the 21 gauge needle through the glistening gray capsule and drew back, my syringe filled with clear fluid: not bile, not blood, not pus. What, then? Urine? Whatever it was, there seemed little danger in draining it, and 600 mL later the cyst was completely deflated. Now, when I grasped the thick capsule and pulled, the cyst rose completely from the abdomen revealing a 1 cm pedicle from the gallbladder. Whatever the underlying cause of this cyst, and despite the fact that it clearly originated from the gallbladder wall, it was not currently communicating with the biliary tract at all. I made a quick decision to remove the gallbladder along with the cyst, in order to prevent recurrence. As I did this, I rehearsed my next interaction with her owners: the heroic surgeon emerging from the operating room with the news that she had achieved the seemingly impossible.

The rest of Petunia's abdomen was an empty shell. Her kidneys were two flattened disks clinging to the retroperitoneum. Her stomach was shrunken and empty, and her spleen a thin wisp barely visible within her omentum. Her jejunum was wriggling in obvious ecstasy following its liberation from the incredible shrinking room, and her bladder was a tiny nut within her pelvic cavity. You could see everything.

Since my journey of discovery in Petunia's abdomen, I have used the "deflation" technique many times: for gallbladders, liver and prostatic abscesses, thymic and branchial cysts, granulomas, and anal sacs.

As an added benefit to the improved visualization that deflation allows *around* a cystic mass, it also allows better investigation of attachments and communications from *inside* the capsule. You can probe and inspect, work out its origin, and where it might be draining to. You can better identify the mucosa lining the cyst (especially if it is surrounded by a lot of fibrous tissue) and be more confident in achieving complete excision.

But, as everything is a balance, you need to recognize the potential downsides to this approach. It is rarely a good idea to cut into a cavity filled with blood, without first establishing there is no ongoing communication with the vascular system (I learned this lesson early, then had to learn it again at the end of my career, as you will see later). Draining and exploring the interior of an abscess will lead to contamination of the surgical site, and must be accompanied by vigorous lavage and institution of appropriate drainage and antibiotics. Finally, if the mass is neoplastic, opening it will cause wound bed contamination and possible local spread. There are several distinct risks in the deflation method.

However, when faced with a mass that might be otherwise inoperable, sometimes those calculated risks are worth taking. I used the deflation technique to help remove an enormous thyroid cyst that was extending deep into the thorax (Figure 2.4), although in retrospect I

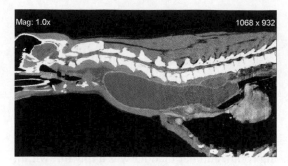

Figure 2.4 Contrast-enhanced CT shows an invasive thyroid cyst extending from the larynx to the heart base in a dog (see also cover photo). Courtesy of the Veterinary Medical Teaching Hospital, School of Veterinary Medicine, UC Davis.

might have done the dog more of a favor had I just marsupialized it, rather than stripping out its entire cervical and thoracic length.

Back in Petunia's abdomen, I was now able to inspect the biliary tree more thoroughly, and it was not an encouraging sight. The remnant of the gallbladder, and the intrahepatic and common bile ducts were thickened and dilated, and I could not convince myself that the opening to the duodenum was patent. My elation about relieving Petunia of her spectacular cyst gave way to concern that said miracle would not actually resolve her spectacular jaundice.

I had a dilemma. If I closed Petunia up now she would certainly be happier as her abdominal organs returned to leading normal lives, but would her bile flow freely? I passed a fine infant feeding tube antegradely into the massively dilated biliary tree. After negotiating the tortuous junction between the cystic and hepatic ducts, it slipped straight into the duodenum. This was promising, but if there were no biliary outflow obstruction, why were the ducts so distended? It seemed hard to explain everything by pressure from the cyst. I had already removed her gallbladder, so no longer had the option of diverting bile flow by performing a cholecysto-duodenostomy. I could probably have anastomosed the distended bile duct to the bowel, but

had never read or seen that procedure. I knew that biliary diversion had its risks, and I didn't know whether it was necessary or not.

Learning point: *you can't always fix everything in one go.*

I began to approach this dilemma from a different perspective.

What if it were *my* bile duct that another surgeon was evaluating? What decision would I want them to make? I decided I would prefer to be given the benefit of the doubt, and only have a diversionary procedure performed if I truly needed it, rather than "just in case."

But a second procedure would be expensive, and if Petunia became progressively more jaundiced she would be a worse anesthetic and surgical candidate, and there were substantial financial implications for the owners. As we will see with many cases in this book, these dilemmas occur frequently in veterinary surgery, and there is not always a textbook answer.

In Petunia's case, I decided to give her biliary tract the benefit of the doubt. In order to hasten her recovery, and provide a mechanism for postoperative evaluation, I placed a small Foley catheter through her right lateral abdominal wall and into the dilated bile duct, thereby creating a choledochostomy. This enabled us to drain bile, hasten resolution of Petunia's jaundice, possibly reduce the pain of biliary distention, and also perform a positive contrast study of the bile duct when she was up and about. I had clearly forgotten our struggles to get a plain abdominal X-ray prior to surgery when dreaming up this particular goal!

My next dilemma was Petunia's paper-thin abdominal wall. It seemed likely to tear even when grasped with forceps, let alone hold sutures for the length of time required for wound healing in a patient who was so systemically compromised. Knowing Petunia had a number of risk factors for poor wound healing, I used a suture material that would not be absorbed too quickly, an interrupted suture pattern in the linea alba, a secure subcutaneous layer, and planned to leave the skin sutures in for a lengthy period of time; at least two weeks, and preferably three.

Petunia was one of the greatest "gift cases" of my residency. She didn't look back after surgery, her jaundice rapidly resolved, when we injected radiographic contrast material into her bile duct it flowed promptly into the duodenum, giving me confidence to remove the Foley catheter two weeks after surgery. Her owners were delighted, and I started to develop a reputation around town as a surgeon who would give things a try when others would not.

"We're just so grateful that you didn't give up on her," said Petunia's owners.

And so was I.

3

The Friday Night Special

Or Why Do Patients Become Critical Just Before the Weekend?

In the previous chapter I wrote about my "first principles" approach to some abdominal cases early in my career, and I will share more of those fledgling experiences and challenges in later chapters. But for now, let's fast forward to the other end of my career, when I was a professor of surgery at the University of California, Davis, and work through some more recent clinical dilemmas using the benefit of many years' experience.

It was Friday evening and we had squeezed two surgery Faculty with their respective residents, six students, and an international visitor into the soft tissue surgery office, for wrap-up rounds. In these debriefing chats, the tradition was to run through details of the cases we had seen during the week and find out if anyone had unanswered questions. At the end, I asked everyone to choose their "highlight" for the week. This might be something they had learned, something that took them by surprise, or maybe a "light bulb" moment when they understood a concept for the first time.

Finding the foxtail in a cervical abscess was a popular one, or being allowed to wield the LigaSure™ when removing a splenic tumor. Seeing the linear foreign body cat start eating again always lifted the spirits. It could seem a long time between Monday and Friday, and this was a nice way to remind ourselves of all the cases we had seen during the week, the things we had learned, and the difference we had made to patients and clients.

In an ideal world, activity in our service wound down late on a Friday afternoon. We would wheel the last patient from the operating room, change the last bandage, submit the last path sample, and sit down to pat ourselves on the back.

My highlight of this particular week was being able to find an ovarian remnant by means of laparoscopy.

Our first year resident, Steph, waxed lyrical about the enormous polyp she had plucked from a cat's nasopharynx.

"Bingo!" With an exaggerated flourish of her hand, she replayed the glorious moment the polyp came free. Her student made a loud sucking noise and we all laughed.

I checked the clock; it was 5:05, a very respectable time to finish, and on such a high note.

"Let's get our orders done," I said. "Make sure everyone is settled down for the night ..."

The top of a head appeared at the small window in the office door, closed so our laughter would not drift down to the waiting room. I watched the head bob and eyes appear as a short person went on tippy toes to peek through the relatively high window. There was only one short person likely to need our attention at this hour on a Friday.

Our surgery tech, Caleb, opened the door and the internal medicine resident tumbled in, looking sheepish.

"Ye..hus?" Part question, part comment; everyone uttered it in unison.

"I don't suppose you're here to invite us for a beer at the Irish pub?" I said.

She shook her head. "I've got a septic abdomen."

Pitfalls in Veterinary Surgery, First Edition. Edited by Geraldine B. Hunt.
© 2017 John Wiley & Sons, Inc. Published 2017 by John Wiley & Sons, Inc.

"How uncomfortable for you."

"It's in ultrasound at the moment."

"Go!" I said to Steph, which was unnecessary because she was already half out the door on her way to diagnostic imaging.

"The good old Friday night special!" our other resident, Andrea, explained to the students. "Never fails!"

"I'm always nervous when we get to 5 or 6 o'clock on a Friday and it hasn't arrived yet," I added.

It was worse than that; I began trawling our computerized medical database on Thursday to see what crazy cases were booked in for appointments on Friday, or who was already in hospital that might suddenly become emergent in about 24 hours.

The Friday night special was so reliable we took "orders" around mid-afternoon.

"What do you want to see?" I would ask the students.

They were always enthusiastic, even though it would mean a late night or possibly no sleep at all.

"GDV!"

"Hemoabdomen!"

"Intestinal foreign body!"

"Infected adrenal tumor!" Every group has one of *those* students.

Unfortunately, the Friday night special is not usually the type of case that students want to see. It is often esoteric, it is usually complicated, and it is frequently a long time getting into surgery.

Sometimes it arrives in the emergency room on the dot of 5, sometimes it takes the form of a phone call to say the owners are on their way. Friday peak hour is a terrible time on the Interstate 80; the weekend traffic fighting its way up to Lake Tahoe for skiing in winter, camping and fishing in summer.

The waiting is the worst part, as the evening drags on and the promised patient still hasn't arrived.

"We're caught in traffic."

"Our car's broken down."

"We've just left Portland (Oregon) and should be there in about eight hours."

One Friday afternoon I was informed that a cat with bilateral ureteral obstructions was currently on a small plane en route from Anchorage, Alaska. The Friday night special's medical complexities are rivaled only by its logistical ones.

The students and I raised the septic abdomen's record on the computer and started reading.

Bose was an eight-year-old Standard Poodle with a history of hip dysplasia which had led to progressively worsening osteoarthritis. I had already scanned his file during my Thursday afternoon stalking and could see where this was heading. I was about to ask the students what connection they saw between the dog's lameness and his septic abdomen, when another face appeared at the door. Actually it was two: the Emergency intern and her attending Faculty member.

"Do you know there is a septic abdomen floating around?"

"We're on it," I said. "Steph just went down to ultrasound to check it out."

"Great! We'll let Anesthesia know," the pair grabbed a pink anesthetic request form from the pigeonhole next to the door and swept away.

It had been a busy week and we were all tired, so it took the students a few minutes to find the connection between Bose's owners' decision to increase the dose of his non-steroidal anti-inflammatory medication and the development of a suspected leak in his gastrointestinal tract.

"Perforated gastric ulcer," they concluded.

"Seems likely," I agreed. We now knew that the sonographer had identified turbid fluid in the peritoneal cavity, tapped it and sent it to Cytology, who confirmed the presence of degenerate neutrophils and intracellular bacteria.

"We consider intracellular bacteria an absolute indication for immediate surgery," I told the students. "There are not many: pus, air, and bile, basically."

"How about blood?"

"What about urine?"

"Not without further tests or treatment," I replied.

Steph still hadn't returned from ultrasound, so we continued discussing acute surgical crises of the abdomen. With a little prompting, the students decided that – faced with a hemoabdomen – they would check coagulation status, try to rule out a history of trauma, gauge the patient's response to fluid resuscitation, and – if at all possible – perform an abdominal ultrasound before leaping into surgery. They had started asking great questions about identifying the site of leakage in a hypothetical patient with uroabdomen when a third group of people arrived.

This time, it was the Community Medicine Faculty, Dr. Julie Meadows, with two students. "We have a septic abdomen …"

"I know," I interrupted. "Steph is in ultrasound with it at the moment, and ER has submitted an Anesthesia request."

"Oh," Julie seemed taken aback, but pleased nonetheless. "How did they find out about it?"

Word travels fast in a veterinary teaching hospital, so I wasn't surprised. Steph reappeared with an update. "Gas tracking in the wall of the stomach. They suspect a perforated ulcer."

The students high-fived one another.

The ER intern swung past and said, "We're going to get the septic abdomen on fluids right now and Anesthesia is ready to start as soon as possible."

"Seems like everything is under control," I said happily.

Julie frowned, "I haven't got permission from the owner yet; we wanted to run it past you first."

"I spoke to the owners already," Steph chipped in. She was very organized. "They've paid their deposit and are on their way home."

Sometimes you get lucky with the Friday night special, but you have to move fast, as there seems to be a golden window in the late afternoon when everyone is invested in moving things along quickly and you can sneak in before the day shift finishes.

Julie opened her mouth, presumably to comment on the way her case had been hijacked, but was interrupted by my phone. It was Radiology.

"We've got a great septic abdomen down here! I think you'll want to check out the ultrasound before you cut it."

"Steph was just down there," I said. "Perforated gastric ulcer?"

"No, that was Bose, the Standard Poodle."

"Huh?" I had a growing feeling that everything was not quite as "under control" as I had thought.

"What did you find in his abdomen?"

I had a reputation for being a fast surgeon, but not quite that fast. "We haven't started him yet. Which patient are you talking about?"

"The Maine Coon."

With a sinking feeling, I turned to Dr. Meadows, who was conferring with her students just outside the door, "Is your patient a Maine Coon?"

She shook her head. "Alaskan Malamute." She indicated a sad-looking dog squatting in the corridor and said to her student, "Sophia, can you give Dr. Hunt the run-down on Carmine?"

Sophia opened a thick paper file and I put up my hand to temporarily stop her.

"What …" my voice broke as I returned to the phone and the waiting radiologist. "What have you found in the Maine Coon?"

"Cholangitis, bile peritonitis, and a ruptured hepatic abscess."

"Go!" I said to the second surgery resident, but Andrea was already on her way.

I looked at Dr. Meadows and her student, Sophia. Having run out of surgery residents to filter this information overload, I felt escalating panic as Sophia detailed Carmine's history; starting with his treatment three years previously for bacterial pyoderma.

Decoding my non-verbal signals, Julie jumped in, "We think he has an infected adrenal tumor."

I resisted a glance at the smart-arse student who had ordered just such a case, but did wonder whether he had been stalking the medical records before rounds.

"Have you told Anesthesia?" I asked faintly.

So how, and why, did these three patients become Friday night surgical specials?

Bose had been in hospital since Thursday morning with lethargy and vomiting, but his owners had only just agreed to further diagnostic testing in light of the fact that he wasn't responding to conservative management with intravenous fluids, antiemetics, and an H2 receptor blocker.

Jazzy, the Maine Coon, had been referred through Emergency from a local practitioner, with a very similar history after conservative management of suspected cholangiohepatitis.

Carmine, who arguably had the most chronic disease, was actually the only peracute patient, having been normal this morning apart from his chronic polyuria (PU), polydipsia (PD), and panting, which the owners had ascribed to the extreme heat of summer. He refused lunch and by afternoon tea (Carmine and his owners let few meal opportunities slip by) he was lethargic and unwilling to walk.

My jaded reflection on how we came to find ourselves in this predicament was interrupted by Carrie, from the Anesthesia Faculty, with a fist full of pink request forms. "Who do you want first?"

We often have to triage, and it is particularly difficult on a Friday night when some patients are in hospital, some are caught in traffic, some owners aren't sure they want to sign the estimate, some need resuscitation before they are stable for surgery, and many of them don't yet have a definitive diagnosis. Being forced to triage is a good stimulus for us to carefully, honestly evaluate the indications and need for surgery (or any other form of treatment, for that matter), rather than making a knee-jerk reaction. Then, assuming that surgery is actually the best option for a given patient, my approach is usually to start with the one who is closest to the operating room. I have been burned too often by holding other cases while we waited for the one "on the way." Another factor to consider is our goal in performing surgery on this patient, at this particular time. We might all agree that emergency surgery is required to save its life, but is that all we are trying to do?

Carmine had a retroperitoneal abscess surrounding a mass that looked like it was effacing the adrenal gland. With his history of PU/PD and panting, it seemed likely his underlying problem was a cortisol-producing tumor. But that wasn't the reason he had been brought to us. He was sitting in the corridor outside the surgery office because he was now acutely sick, with an abscess that needed draining.

Did we know anything about his tumor: its blood supply, its invasiveness, its hormone production? No.

Did we know whether it was resectable, or what the physiologic consequences of removing it would be? No.

So we had to decide on a plan. The natural thing would be to say, *He has an infected adrenal tumor, so let's operate to remove it and drain his abscess.*

But this is a complex surgery, made doubly difficult by the infection and unknown amount of fibrosis resulting from chronic inflammation. A CT angiogram would provide more information about vascularity, local invasion, and prognosis, but, even then, without further testing we couldn't be sure whether it was an adrenal tumor or an inflammatory mass resulting from chronic retroperitoneal inflammation, possibly even a migrating foreign body.

Carmine's urgent need was for his abscess to be drained. Working up and devising a strategy for treating his periadrenal mass was not urgent. So our primary goal for Carmine was to keep him alive to allow further diagnostics.

I verbalized my thought processes regarding the other cases.

"With Jazzy, the Maine Coon, we know she has a hepatic abscess that has presumably ruptured. We suspect it is caused by ascending cholangiohepatitis, and she possibly also has a perforation of the biliary tract. Draining the abscess would treat her emergent problem, but her suspected bile leak is also urgent, so should really be addressed at the same time if possible. Our goal with her is to treat the abscess, but also to resolve the anatomic issue causing the leak and stabilize her to permit further medical treatment of her suspected cholangitis.

Bose has become a Friday night special because his stomach is perforated, and our goal for him is clearly to identify and repair the source of the leak. However, he is currently more stable than either of the others."

The rule for after-hours cases was that, regardless of their level of experience or confidence, residents had to call their Faculty supervisors in three situations: if the patient was septic, if the biliary tree was involved, or if they were going to enter the chest. So it was probably no accident that Faculty – or at least this one – prioritized those patients as the evening marched on.

"Let's get started on Jazzy," I decided. Self-interest aside, I justified this on the basis that prepping a cat and performing abdominal exploration was almost always going to be faster than for a dog, and hopefully by the time we had Jazzy under control our next patient would be just about to hit the table.

I turned back to Julie and her students, working on medical records at our computer while waiting to get a word in.

"What I am hearing," she said, "is that Carmine needs to be stabilized surgically as soon as possible, and once that is done, he needs further diagnostics, which would probably include a CT, to work out whether his adrenal mass can be treated."

She turned to her students. "So what should we do next?"

"An abdominal explore."

"Before that."

"Antibiotics?"

"Even before that."

"Stabilize with IV fluids?"

"While we're doing that."

One student, quiet so far, raised her hand. "Talk to the owners and see whether they are prepared to spend the money for emergency surgery tonight, knowing that it is just the beginning, and we don't know Carmine's prognosis until we work out what the mass is."

Julie and I traded a smile. Who said that students could not learn from complex cases? The trick is to break the complex cases down into simple concepts; not because the students can't cope with complex – most of them are smarter than I am – but because until we break out the simple concepts, it is extremely hard to devise an objective strategy, and almost impossible to discuss it effectively with the owners.

My smile faded when Carmine's student said his owners had gone home to wait for news.

"Where do they live?" I asked.

"West Sac. But they said they would come right back once we had some results."

Fortunately, West Sacramento was only 12 miles away and this was a conversation I would prefer to have in person.

"I'll call them right now," said the student.

Jazzy was in the operating room ready for an incision within an hour of her pink form being submitted. Her abdomen was filled with bile-tinged serosanguinous fluid and her liver was discolored and enlarged. It appeared she did have a case of rampant cholangitis and an abscess had formed around her necrotic gallbladder. Despite the spectacular state of her abdomen, it was relatively straightforward to remove the gallbladder, drain and debride the hepatic abscess, and collect biopsies for histopathology and microbiology. As we were lavaging her peritoneal cavity, I enquired about the status of our other patients.

"The stomach is a go," said the OR tech.

"How about the adrenal dog?"

"I haven't heard anything."

I left my very capable surgery resident, Andrea, to place Jazzy's closed suction drain and scrubbed out. I found Dr. Meadows and her students in the corridor between the OR and ICU.

"What's happening?"

"Carmine's owners have just arrived," they replied. It was over two hours since they had left West Sacramento to "come straight back in" so I was surprised; there must have been a pile-up on the I-80.

"Shall we speak to them together?" This would save time, which was becoming more critical as Carmine's sepsis worsened and my grumbling stomach reminded me it was well past dinnertime.

Carmine's entire family had come to visit. Carmine himself was in good body condition, and it quickly became evident the trait was hereditary. They were an impressive biomass, especially when crammed into one of the small consulting rooms we termed a "fishbowl." All five were holding McDonald's thick shakes.

"It's getting late," said Carmine's Dad, "so we thought we'd eat before we came in."

The teenage daughter handed over a quarter pounder and fries. It smelled good.

How thoughtful, they brought something for us too.

"For Carmine," she said.

All of which suggested that they weren't totally clear on the gravity of the situation.

Carmine did not go to surgery that night. Instead, we drained the abscess sonographically, submitted samples for microbiology, and started him on antibiotics. His owners weren't up for one surgery, let alone two. He recovered sufficiently to leave hospital, after which we lost him to follow-up. We never did work out whether he had a true adrenal mass, or just a wad of fibrous tissue surrounding a migrating foreign body.

Our month continued with a theme of sepsis, and each of the following two Friday evenings served up remarkably similar cases, whose major presenting complaints were "fever and swelling."

We were alerted to Tebow on Thursday afternoon when Connie, our duty tech, received a call from Reception.

"We have a client on the phone whose dog urgently needs surgery. Can they make an appointment for tomorrow morning?"

"What's the problem?" asked Connie.

"He has a leaking abdomen."

Connie shot me a glance. "Leaking abdomen" could mean any number of things, few of which were good.

"They should come in through Emergency," she said to Reception. "As soon as possible."

The next we knew of Tebow was when ER came to us on Friday evening and said, "We may have a surgery case for you."

Actually, what really happened was that just as we wrapped up rounds after a particularly stressful week, the ER resident peeked around the corner as if he expected to be shot.

"There is *nothing* you could tell us right now that would be welcome," snapped a member of our team who shall remain nameless.

He winced.

"We *especially* don't want to hear that you have a cat with ureteral obstructions."

He grinned with relief, "No."

"Oh. Well, that's alright then."

"It's kind of a weird one, though," he said.

Tebow was a seven-year-old Boxer cross who had received extensive veterinary attention at another clinic for a suspected body wall abscess. He was lethargic and febrile, with a painful swelling extending from his right axilla, along his chest wall and into his cranial abdomen. Tebow's history was complicated by the fact that he had presented to his regular vet about two weeks previously for vomiting and anorexia and, after failing to respond to empirical treatment, had undergone abdominal exploration. The abdominal explore had been unremarkable except for some thickening around the pylorus, so the vet took a serosal biopsy and performed a prophylactic incisional gastropexy.

Tebow never recovered completely from surgery; he continued to vomit intermittently and the subcutaneous swelling became noticeable over the last five days. There was concern that his gastropexy or biopsy sites had perforated into his body wall, leading to the "leaking abdomen" enquiry of the previous night.

The question on everyone's lips, as Friday afternoon turned into Friday evening was, "Does he need surgery?"

Tebow smelled. And I don't mean that he smelled literally septic, or necrotic. There was an odor to his story that hinted at some underlying problem of which we were currently unaware, like a faint smell of rot drifting down from the attic.

Tebow's student told us the owners were expecting us to "open him up" again.

"Here's the question," I replied. "What are we going to 'open up' and why?"

Were we going to open up his abdomen and explore the pyloric antrum? Were we going to open up the swelling to try to drain an abscess?

"Do we have any evidence that he has an infection?" I asked.

"Swelling, pain, fever, heat."

"I agree we have inflammation. But do we have infection?"

"I don't know."

"How could we find out?"

The students chose a full blood count and a fine needle aspiration (FNA).

The sonographers had been there before us and identified a massive amount of subcutaneous edema. In the absence of a fluid pocket in the subcutis, or within the peritoneal cavity, they had aspirated the swelling in a number of areas.

"What did the cytology show?" I asked.

"Inconclusive."

Applying the term "inconclusive" to a cytology result always bothers me.

"Do you mean 'inconclusive' in that they didn't give the disease a name, or inconclusive in that it wasn't a good sample?"

We read through the cytology report. The pathologist had seen red blood cells, some normal leukocytes, and a lot of fat, but little else. Either the aspirates were not representative of the underlying problem, or we were not dealing with bacterial cellulitis. Couple that with the sonographer's failure to locate any fluid pockets, and it was hard to know how we were going to help Tebow with surgery, tonight at least.

After explaining to Tebow's owners that we could not recommend surgery in the absence of any discrete disease process to go after, we left him in ER's capable hands. They treated him symptomatically over the weekend, and on Monday they performed another ultrasound, which now identified several masses in his axilla. A guided FNA yielded poorly differentiated mast cells. In retrospect, it all made sense. Tebow had an aggressive mast cell tumor; histamine release led to gastrointestinal ulceration with resultant vomiting and inappetance. As the tumors in his axilla grew, they caused local inflammation, and hence the spreading edema. Tebow's prognosis was very poor,

and although we were not able to help him with surgery, at least I was happy we had spared him any more unnecessary procedures.

Fast forward almost a week to Mignon. We were alerted to this potential Friday night special by an excited ER student who came to tell her friend – currently on the surgery rotation – of a robust three-and-a-half-year-old Labrador with a one-week history of "back pain" and increasing lethargy. Over the past two to three days, Mignon had developed progressive swelling of his left thorax and flank which was now extending into his inguinal area. The swelling was hot and painful, he resented palpation, and he was febrile.

"Ah," the students said sagely. "Mast cell tumor."

"Not so quick," I said, knowing that in Mignon's case, the FNA of his subcutaneous swelling had yielded degenerate neutrophils and intracellular bacteria.

"Cool," they said. "Shall we tell Anesthesia?"

Now we had a different dilemma. It appeared Mignon had rampant bacterial cellulitis. Everyone was desperate to fix him, and it was Thursday evening, and who knew how badly things might deteriorate if we left him overnight? But did that make him a surgical case?

California being the foxtail capital of the world, we thought the most likely explanation was migrating plant material, but the sonographers could find neither a foreign body nor an organized abscess.

Mignon's owners expressed the hope that we could just cut out the infected tissue. Had we been confident of a diagnosis of necrotizing fasciitis, that is exactly what we should have done, but Mignon's swelling was now affecting one third of his body – so where to start and where to finish? With nothing discrete to go after, it was hard to get excited about surgery as his best option.

We agreed the ideal approach would be to send Mignon for CT in the hope of finding the underlying focus of infection. But there was a real chance CT would not identify anything surgical, in which case the owners were up for the costs of anesthesia and imaging, without influencing the treatment plan substantially. If we found a deep abscess cavity we could drain it, but was late Thursday night really the best time to embark on a foxtail explore of the retroperitoneal space? The decision-making was rather similar to that for Tebow. Mignon was in our emergency room because he had a generalized soft tissue infection, and until it turned into an abscess any surgical intervention was arbitrary, at best.

When the owners were given all these options, they chose to let us treat Mignon conservatively with supportive treatment and antibiotics, in the hope that we could either resolve his infection or at least buy time until the site declared itself.

One issue that weighs on our minds when deciding when to take a case to surgery is the impending weekend. There's the thought that it is better to get it "over and done with" because the weekend is, after all, the weekend. But I can think of few circumstances where it is better to operate on a stable patient late in the evening than during the day, even if the following day falls on a weekend.

Mignon received his antimicrobials, analgesics, and intravenous fluids; his swelling and fever subsided marginally. Less than 48 hours later, a flash ultrasound of his thoracoabdominal area showed that his abscess had finally declared itself. Instead of a Friday night special, Mignon had become a Saturday morning hangover.

As Mignon was waking up in the post-anesthetic recovery ward, a tie-over bandage sutured to the open wound on his side, on the other side of the Pacific the Fitzgerald family were enjoying that classic Australian Sunday evening meal: the lamb roast. Mr. Fitzgerald carved slices from the leg and served them to everyone around the table.

"Stop it!" cried Katie, who was 10.

"It wasn't me!" snapped her older sister.

"Frankie's licking my leg!" said Katie.

"Nice job, Frankie," said her sister approvingly.

"Frankie, stop it," Mrs. Fitzgerald instructed.

Frankie, the four-year-old Staffy cross, crept back from under the table and sat in the middle of the kitchen with an "if you insist" expression.

"He's hungry," said Katie.

"No feeding the dog at the table," said Mrs. Fitzgerald.

They passed roast vegetables and gravy around and everyone served themselves. They took no more notice of Frankie, who crept back between Katie and her big sister and sat with his mouth slightly open in the hope that some succulent tidbit might fall from their plates.

On Monday morning, we changed Mignon's bandage. His wound looked healthy and the amount of discharge was markedly decreased. We had not located the suspected foxtail, but we had drained a satisfying amount of pus from the abscess at surgery and Mignon was looking better each day. Sometime in the next couple of days we would repair the wound and place a closed suction drain.

That same evening, the Fitzgeralds sat down to the traditional Monday dinner – usually eaten the day following a lamb roast: shepherd's pie.

"You've got a good appetite this week, Katie," said Mrs. Fitzgerald. Usually fussy, the 10-year-old dispatched her first serving and asked for seconds.

Her sister, surreptitiously exchanging texts with her boyfriend, saw Frankie licking the floor next to Katie's chair, but decoding Peter's emojis was more important, so she said nothing.

After dinner, Mrs. Fitzgerald put the lamb bone, which she had stripped of meat for the shepherd's pie, into the garbage bin. Katie's sister was called upon to take out the garbage, about which she would normally complain bitterly, but this time it afforded her the opportunity to have a quick smoke behind the garden shed. She dumped the garbage bag in the general vicinity of the bin, and lit an illicit cigarette.

The next morning, as she raced out to catch the school bus, she noticed the shredded garbage bag, its contents strewn around like debris from a well-focused tornado. But she was more worried about the damning evidence of cigarette butts scattered amongst the table scraps. She swept it all up and dumped it into the trash can.

Around lunchtime on Tuesday, Clarissa – a first year Medicine resident – called by.

"I have a case coming from Ventura," she said. "Pancreatitis. I'm just giving you a heads-up because it has biliary obstruction."

"No worries." I am always far more polite early in the week, after the Monday morning rush is over but before our surgery schedule is full, and especially so with a case that hasn't even arrived yet.

When she did arrive, "Ginger" Rogers' mucous membranes were delightfully color coordinated with her name; she was a bright orange–yellow.

The Medicine student introduced herself to the owners in order to take a history and do a physical exam. She appeared back in the rounds room almost immediately. "She won't let me touch her."

"Ginger?"

"No, Mrs. Rogers."

We all have clients who "don't want students touching their pet." Sometimes this extends to residents, or even to anyone who is not a boarded specialist. It can be quite hard to persuade some people that we don't intend to leave their pets alone to be butchered by people who don't know what they're doing. I mean, whose best interests would that serve?

In this case, Mrs. Rogers was prepared to speak to the resident, in order to explain her requirements for Ginger.

"She's impossible to reason with," said Clarissa, almost an hour later; flopped on a chair in the soft tissue surgery office.

Clarissa and I had already discussed the possible options and outcomes for Ginger, and developed a strategy that only included surgical intervention if her biliary obstruction did not resolve with medical management of her pancreatitis. It seemed so clear to us; why didn't Mrs. Rogers get it?

"She just wants surgery," said Clarissa.

A student huffed. "Why did she come here if she isn't going to take our advice?"

Channeling Dr. Julie Meadows, from whom I was learning a more compassionate approach to doctoring, I said, "Let's look at it from her point of view. Why do you think she is behaving this way?"

Please, no allusions to female dogs or bovines, I thought.

"How would you be feeling if you were her?"

"Frustrated," one student offered. "Ginger is sick and she's traveled all this way."

"Distrustful."

"Scared," said another.

"All that, and I think she just wants her dog to be made better," I said, "and in her mind, that is going to require surgery. So, if we try to persuade her against surgery, it's tantamount to telling her that we aren't trying to cure Ginger."

"Somehow," said Clarissa, with a new lease of life after venting her frustration, "we have to convince her we are all trying for the same thing. Let's go talk to her again." As she left the room though, she turned back and said, "But keep Ginger on your radar just in case! If her bilirubin goes up any further, we should probably consider a stent."

We had a "radar" column on the white board in the surgery office, so for the rest of that week, Ginger was on our list without actually being scheduled.

It was Tuesday night in the Fitzgerald household.

"Where's Frankie?" asked Mrs. Fitzgerald.

"In the garden," said Katie.

After raiding the trash bag early that morning, Frankie had chewed on his newfound lamb femur for most of the day, and then licked every remnant of marrow from the splintered diaphysis. Virtually as they were speaking, he sniffed around on the ground, picked up the last fragment of cartilage, and swallowed it.

"Ew! Gross!" said Katie's sister as the dog trotted back into the house, trailing ropes of pearly saliva.

"Go to bed, Frankie," Mrs. Fitzgerald instructed. Frankie was the only family member who still responded to this command, so he dutifully but reluctantly crept into Katie's bedroom.

The evening was peaceful until Katie retired to her room, flopped onto her beanbag to watch *Dancing with the Stars* and howled as she entered a gelatinous pile of half-digested lamb, bone splinters, and grass.

Each day for the remainder of that week, we stalked VMACS to see what Ginger's bilirubin was doing. For the first two days, it hovered around 15. At least it wasn't going up, and Clarissa had worked some psychological magic with Mrs. Rogers, who had agreed to try to science rather than the scalpel. We almost considered erasing Ginger from the "radar."

By Wednesday morning, it was clear to everyone in the Fitzgerald house that Frankie was sick. Banished to his outside run after throwing up all over Katie's bedroom, he spent most of the night gagging loudly outside the window. By morning, he seemed a little more settled, but he crept out to see the kids off to school without his usual bounce, and his tail barely raised a wag.

"If you aren't looking better when I come back from tennis," Mrs. Fitzgerald said, "I am taking you up to the vet."

Lunchtime brought a very sad-looking dog. He was almost constantly drooling, hiccuping, and retching sporadically without bringing anything up.

The local vets determined him to be nauseous and dehydrated.

"Leave him with us. We'll put him on a drip. Hopefully, he just has a case of garbage guts and he'll recover once his stomach has a chance to rest."

It was a subdued night in the Fitzgerald house. They passed the evening on Twitter, watching *The X Factor*, and reading *Game of Thrones* before falling asleep early to make up for the night before.

Thursday was the day that Ginger's bilirubin suddenly rose again and she went back on the surgical radar. But although her bilirubin was higher, she looked clinically better. She was more comfortable and she had even started eating a little. Although we had agreed we would consider surgery if her jaundice worsened, it was hard to make that call in light of the fact she seemed to be improving. We had another interdisciplinary conference, and Clarissa had another lengthy discussion with the owner. We would give her another day and see what happened. I was beginning to have serious misgivings. For a change, it seemed we were slowly but surely creating our own Friday night special.

Frankie was happier after his intravenous fluids, but still not himself. He continued to salivate, and although his retching had subsided with a couple of doses of maropitant, he turned his head whenever food was offered. This seemed more extreme than your normal case of garbage intoxication.

"Pancreatitis or a bowel obstruction seem the most likely explanations," the vet said to Katie and Mrs. Fitzgerald when they visited on Thursday afternoon. "If he has a bowel obstruction he might need surgery."

Oh no! thought Katie, scared at what that might mean.

Oh no! thought Mrs. Fitzgerald, scared at what that might cost.

"Ideally, we should do some blood work and an abdominal ultrasound. But the radiologist doesn't visit until tomorrow."

"Maybe Frankie will be better tomorrow?"

"Maybe, but if he needs surgery we don't want to delay. How about we run some basic bloods and take an abdominal X-ray?"

Frankie's blood work was unremarkable, which the vets told Mrs. Fitzgerald was good because it ruled out disease of the liver or kidney. His abdominal radiograph was also unremarkable, with no obstructive pattern or obvious foreign body. Frankie had bought himself another day of observation.

Late Thursday night, though, Frankie was febrile. He was started on antibiotics. By Friday morning, he was drooling and retching uncontrollably. Later that day the Fitzgeralds authorized an abdominal ultrasound. It didn't show anything out of the ordinary. There was some discussion about taking Frankie straight to surgery for an abdominal explore anyway, but it was hard to make that call in the absence of an obvious lesion. Nonetheless, Frankie was getting progressively worse despite treatment. In the mid-afternoon, Frankie developed a soft cough, and began breathing heavily. With this progressive deterioration in Frankie's condition, and the weekend looming, the vet on duty picked up the telephone.

Lunchtime Friday, on the other hand, brought some excellent news for Ginger Rogers and for the rest of us. Her bilirubin level had dived to below 10! She looked bright when walking outside, and her appetite was coming back. An abdominal ultrasound showed that her common bile duct was decreasing in diameter. Her biliary obstruction was resolving. What a close shave.

We finished our Friday afternoon rounds, and my highlight for the week was the ongoing descent of Ginger's bilirubin. Despite a growing sense of unease as the witching hour of 6 p.m. approached, there were no sheepish faces at our door, and we finished the day. I packed up my things, put on my cycling gear, and walked down

the steps to the back door of the hospital. It was my last day after three weeks on clinic, and another Faculty surgeon, Phil Mayhew, was after-hours back up. I was off duty!

As I unlocked my bike chain, I heard the hospital PA system, *"ER tech to reception STAT!"*

Some species of emergency had arrived. I smiled. Not because a poor pet and its owner were in desperate straits, but because our hospital never slept. I might be leaving and going home for the day, but someone else's day was just beginning. The cycle would go on long after I retired as a veterinarian. But I would have had a major role in training many of those clinicians, and they would expand their knowledge and their own horizons, always advancing the profession and making a greater and greater difference to their non-human charges. And that was a very rewarding thought.

Half way across the world, in another specialist center, Frankie Fitzgerald was carried into reception. He was dehydrated and dyspneic, and his owners were in tears. Their Friday night special had arrived.

4

Between a Rock and a Hard Place

When to Refer and What Do You Do When Referral Is Not an Option?

There are many reasons for patients to be referred. With Frankie Fitzgerald it was an act of desperation. Here was a young, previously healthy patient who continued to deteriorate despite his vets' best efforts. They did not know what was causing Frankie's problem, but it became clear he was going to die without assistance.

In the previous chapter, we saw numerous patients that were referred as a last resort. But most specialists would say that, given a choice, they prefer to see the patients before they became emergent and I am sure that most vets prefer to send patients off before things get out of control.

Referral is a complex situation, with multiple factors in play, so it isn't surprising there is no "one size fits all" approach. Everyone involved has a perspective: the referring veterinarian, their boss or practice manager, the owner (and their various family members), the specialist receiving the referral, their client services manager, and so on. And in trying to fulfil expectations of those various stakeholders we have the overarching challenge of attempting to advocate effectively and compassionately for the patient.

Viewing Frankie's case from the perspectives of the various stakeholders (not necessarily in order of importance), and seeing as I am the one writing this, let's start with the specialist to whom he was referred.

This dog, which is at death's door, turns up at the very end of the week. There is no working diagnosis, and a full blood count and chemistry panel from the day before yesterday, an abdominal radiograph, and an abdominal ultrasound yield no clues. At least Frankie helped by demonstrating that his most acute problem was his inability to breathe. Pulse oximetry showed his oxygen saturation to be 85: right on the scary part of the curve. Frankie was placed on intranasal oxygen in ICU while they gathered a history and worked out a plan.

Viewing Frankie's case from the perspective of his owner (in this case, Mrs. Fitzgerald, as the family representative): she took Frankie to the vet because he was sick and not getting better. They were given a range of possibilities, the most likely being a case of "garbage guts" which would likely resolve with fasting and symptomatic treatment. However, Frankie continued to deteriorate despite being given intravenous fluids and other medications.

It was then suggested that they should do blood work and also an abdominal radiograph, both of which were costly and neither of which showed any particular reason for Frankie's ongoing illness.

There was talk of taking Frankie to surgery, but they all agreed that it would be prudent to confirm the nature of the problem first. The trouble was, after paying for a Radiology consultant to come in, the abdominal ultrasound showed nothing spectacular either; leaving them with a situation where Frankie might still need surgery, but they couldn't be absolutely sure. The only thing the tests had added were doubts.

Now Frankie was very sick – in fact he looked like he might be *dying* – and nobody seemed to

Pitfalls in Veterinary Surgery, First Edition. Edited by Geraldine B. Hunt.
© 2017 John Wiley & Sons, Inc. Published 2017 by John Wiley & Sons, Inc.

know what was going on. It was Friday afternoon ... surely everyone would be going home for the weekend soon and then who would be around to look after Frankie? When their vet suggested a chest X-ray, it became clear the dog needed a level of care he was not getting there. With a great deal of trepidation, and after twisting her husband's arm, Mrs. Fitzgerald picked up the phone and called the referral center. They did not have a lot of money to spare, but Frankie was part of their family, and they couldn't see him slowly fading away. Surely someone must be able to find the best medicine for him?

Inspecting Frankie's case from the perspective of the local veterinarian: the dog presented with a history of being fed fatty meat from the dinner table (Katie denied this, but the rest of the family refused to believe her). Mrs. Fitzgerald was reluctant to authorize many (expensive) diagnostic tests if there was a good chance that Frankie would recover with simple conservative management. Frankie's vets, like many others in multi-vet practices around the world, worked an overlapping four-day week, alternating consulting and surgery, which included treatments on hospitalized patients. The vet who examined Frankie on Tuesday was not the same one who evaluated him on Wednesday. And then they swapped again on Thursday. They were busy trying to keep up with the influx of patients through the door, and neither of them had a good handle on Frankie's condition. They were frustrated that none of their diagnostic tests yielded any useful information; getting permission to run tests was a constant struggle, and now they were over their original estimate for diagnosis and treatment. Frankie kept getting sicker and his owners were harder and harder to communicate with. Things were breaking down rapidly, and by Friday afternoon all parties were desperate for resolution. The vets were relieved when they shipped Frankie off to the specialist, but also nervous. What would they find? And could Frankie be saved?

The Fitzgeralds were distraught as they carried Frankie into the specialist center. A technician

came immediately to examine Frankie, and said she would need to take him straight out the back for oxygen treatment. Frankie was whisked away and they were left to wait.

So how did the referral clinician resolve Frankie's situation? Their approach was simple really: ignoring his original complaint for a moment, they started with the most obviously critical current problem and took a chest X-ray. His chest X-ray was highly suggestive of aspiration pneumonia. While the emergency doctor went to speak with the Fitzgeralds, the techs worked on Frankie's anesthesia plan and fired up the endoscope, as Frankie's chest X-ray had also revealed the underlying cause of his illness (Figure 4.1).

When the doctor returned to the waiting room immediately after taking Frankie's X-ray, the Fitzgeralds imagined the worst.

"Is he going to be alright?"

"He has bad aspiration pneumonia. That's why he isn't breathing so well at the moment. It's a lung infection caused by inhaling saliva or food. In his case, probably because of his vomiting."

"Can you treat it?"

"We are giving him oxygen and we'll start him on antibiotics. The good news is, we think we

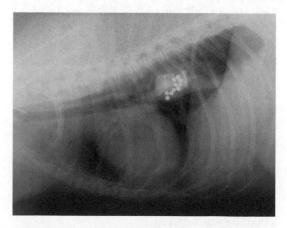

Figure 4.1 Lateral thoracic radiograph in a dog with esophageal foreign body. The dog was fed barium-impregnated polyethylene spheres in an attempt to diagnose the cause of its "vomiting" and suspected intestinal obstruction.

know what's been causing his problems. He has a bone stuck in his esophagus."

"A bone?" Mrs. Fitzgerald knew cooked bones weren't good for dogs. She would never give Frankie a bone. "Where did he get that?"

"He might have got it out of the trash," mumbled Katie's sister.

The relief of finally getting a diagnosis gave way to doubts about the way he had been treated.

"So that what's been causing his problems all along?"

"I don't know for sure, but it would certainly explain it."

There were many unsaid questions right at that moment. They would be discussed later, but right now one was pre-eminent, "Can you save him?"

"We can try."

And fortunately, they did.

Clients like the Fitzgeralds might be forgiven for a jaded view of their experience. After leaving Frankie to get sicker and sicker at one vet, with no meaningful diagnosis or plan, within half an hour of arriving at the specialist center they are told exactly what the diagnosis is, and quickly come to realize that had they known this three days ago, Frankie would not be in this dire condition.

A specialist in referral practice might also have ungenerous thoughts about the patient who arrives, half-dead, just before the weekend, after another vet has messed around with it for three or four days. How much easier would things have been if Frankie had been referred to them on Wednesday morning, before money had been spent on hospitalization, and unnecessary tests, and before he developed aspiration pneumonia because nobody could differentiate regurgitation from vomiting?

As a student, I witnessed rounds in which a veterinarian was savagely criticized for referring a patient with undiagnosed Cushing's disease. I was shocked on two fronts: first, I hadn't even heard of Cushing's disease despite apparently having been lectured on the subject (it was concealed in a lecture on skin disease). Second, if

this was how referring veterinarians were spoken about when they sent cases to the university, I never wanted to refer anything there. Ever.

So let's be generous when we evaluate cases such as Frankie's, and assume that nobody makes mistakes, withholds treatment, or fails to make a diagnosis on purpose. It just happens that way sometimes, and for very good reasons.

After finishing my PhD, while doing a short locum in private practice, I diagnosed a large splenic mass in a Greyhound cross. In Chapter 2 I wrote about tackling Barney, a Labrador with a very similar mass, during my first year of practice. Ironically, with a little more experience under my belt, I began to doubt my ability. I decided to refer the case to Sydney University and sent it off immediately after the consult.

The practice owner was not impressed. He took me aside when he returned from vacation and said, "Why did you send that case out? We can remove a splenic tumor here."

I tried to explain my concerns about whether we could offer a good surgical service in a one-man practice in which the only after-hours monitoring was left to a 16-year-old living in the practice flat while she finished her last year of high school. I failed.

"I would prefer you don't do that again."

I now had two good reasons to be scared about referring a case: criticism from the people to whom I was referring, and criticism from the person for whom I was working. But it is every client's right to be offered referral, or to seek a second opinion, regardless of how trivial the problem seems, so, compelling as those fears might be, they should be the least important factors to consider.

On the flip side, as clinicians who see referrals or second opinions, we should be constantly mindful of how our comments are perceived. This is particular true for universities and practices conducting student rotations. I've learned first-hand how damaging it can be to the relationship with referring veterinarians should that sort of criticism be relayed back, and the impact it has on by-standing students can be enormous.

It is quite conceivable that Mrs. Fitzgerald went back to Frankie's original veterinarian and demanded to know why they could not diagnose an esophageal foreign body after three days when the specialist did it within a few minutes.

Which means that we now have a third major reason to fear referral: criticism from the client themselves.

Considering the main drivers for seeking specialist input, and the turning points in any given case that might prompt referral, let's look back at the stages of Frankie's treatment and see if things could have turned out differently.

Frankie first presented to the local vet with the history that his doting "sister," Katie, had been slipping him pieces of lamb from the family dinner table. His illness followed two meals of roast lamb, so it was a natural assumption that the events were related. After his first presentation to the local vet, it seemed reasonable to treat for the common, and give him some time to recover on his own.

In actuality, though, the owners had already tried that by waiting over 24 hours after Frankie began showing signs before taking him to the vet, in the hope that he would just get better. But that detail got lost in the general flurry of information, and a day of observation turned into two or three.

If we (as primary veterinarians) see a patient that has just begun vomiting, we are unlikely to say, "Let's watch him for 72 hours to see what happens." But that is often what happens when we don't pay attention to the continuity of a case, and we all know how time gets away!

The day after Frankie was admitted to hospital, he was still looking "nauseous" enough to prompt the vet on duty that day to suggest some additional tests, with the objective of ruling out a surgical condition like a bowel obstruction.

Is this a point at which we might refer a case? I think most vets would say no. Removing a peach stone or a marble from the jejunum is within the scope of the majority of practitioners. The dilemma here is when do you feel you have enough information to take a patient to surgery, or perform any other invasive procedure for that matter? Even in a tertiary referral practice we are sometimes pushed to explore a patient before we have a diagnosis. Some of these explorations reveal the diagnosis, others are negative. So the ability to make a diagnosis has a major role in many cases that are referred.

I warn my residents to take a step back if they find themselves planning surgery in order to make a diagnosis, rather than in response to one.

"This could all work out just fine. But it also might not, and then what are you going to do?"

Because it is a little too easy for me, as a specialist working in a tertiary referral center, to prescribe the ideal conditions for performing surgery, when the situation facing a vet in private practice might be far less cut and dried. I have asked my colleagues – Kate Le Bars, who just happens to be my sister, and Dr. Julie Meadows, who has become a close friend – to share their experiences in the next chapters.

It makes sense that confidence in both your diagnosis and your ability to thoroughly explore the patient are major factors in making a decision to operate, as opposed to referring it or seeking a second opinion.

I am always after second opinions. I am lucky enough to have worked with many other clinicians off whom to bounce ideas. I also had brilliant students and highly experienced techs. Anyone with a vested interest in a case can be a useful resource. Frankie's vets may not have had a raft of specialists with whom to confer, but they had one another, and had they "rounded" on Frankie's case; gone through it from the beginning and revisited it objectively, they might have tumbled to the fact that he was actually regurgitating rather than vomiting. They might have taken a chest radiograph in addition to the abdominal one, and the story could have unfolded quite differently.

"Hi, Mrs. Fitzgerald, we have an update on Frankie."

"Oh yes, how is he today?"

"Well, unfortunately he still looks uncomfortable. He doesn't have a bowel obstruction or anything needing surgery in his abdomen. But I talked his case through with my colleagues, and we wondered whether he might be regurgitating because he can't swallow properly, rather than vomiting. So we took a chest X-ray, and we think he has a bone stuck in his esophagus."

"A bone?" Mrs. Fitzgerald knew cooked bones weren't good for dogs. She would never give Frankie a bone. "Where did he get that?"

"I don't know, but maybe he raided the trash?"

"Can you remove it?"

"It's stuck way down inside his chest, so it would be major surgery. But the specialist center up the road has an endoscope, and they might be able to remove it through his mouth."

"Oh that's great news! When can we take him?"

"We can give you a referral straight away. Would you like to us ring and make an appointment for you?"

"Yes, please! Thank you so much!"

Sometimes you do have to step back, regardless of the investment you have made in a particular diagnostic or treatment plan, and take another look at it, from the beginning and with fresh eyes. Allow yourself to consider alternative explanations. Review all the results, not just the ones that support your preferred diagnosis, and pay particular attention to those clues you may have ignored because they were inconvenient. In many of the cases referred to me through the years, that is all I needed to make a breakthrough.

A six-year-old Old English Sheepdog was referred with a three-week history that included an exploratory laparotomy to investigate the cause of his ascites. The explore was negative, and biopsies merely confirmed peritoneal irritation as a result of fluid accumulation. In truth, it is very hard to ever admit to a negative explore. It is far more tempting to find *some* abnormality, even though it might not really explain the signs. At least it provides an opportunity to biopsy something. And hopefully, by the time the negative biopsy result comes back, the patient will have recovered. Sadly, that did not happen this time.

I sent the students out to introduce themselves and start the consult. I paraphrased something I was told by a visiting registrar, Debbie, during my residency many years earlier.

"When you get a complex case, try not to be intimidated. Just start at the beginning and take a thorough history, and do a thorough physical examination."

The students took this on board, and I did not see them for at least half an hour. When they returned, Brian said, "I can't hear his heart properly. I think he has a pericardial effusion."

Surely it couldn't be that easy? Brian went out to bring the dog back to the treatment room while I tried to find my stethoscope that I swore I had last seen in Ward 2. I eventually found it in Radiology, but that wasn't until much later, and long after I had pinched another one that was lying in the treatment room.

Brian was right; this dog did have muffled heart sounds. A chest radiograph and a flash ultrasound revealed a large fluid accumulation in his pericardium (Figure 4.2). I was delighted, but I also knew that when I met the owners to update them I was about to play out the referring vet's worst nightmare: the virtually instantaneous diagnosis of a problem that had completely escape them. And worse, in trying to find an answer, they had needlessly performed an invasive and expensive procedure that could easily have done a lot more harm than good. When I spoke with the referring vet later that day, he explained that he had done the exploratory

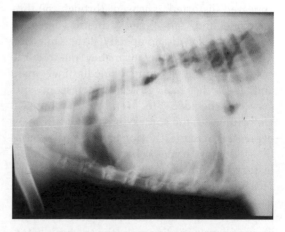

Figure 4.2 Lateral thoracic radiograph (showing pericardial effusion) in a dog following exploratory laparotomy for ascites.

laparotomy in response to a cytology report showing "angry" mesothelial cells in the abdominal fluid.

"I really was expecting to find cancer," he said.

I have found a mesothelioma diagnosis to be very elusive. Few cases with mesothelioma will exfoliate obviously neoplastic cells, and many patients with ascites from other causes show signs of mesothelial activation. I would never take a patient to surgery based purely on the presence of strange-looking mesothelial cells.

But I didn't say that to the vet in so many words; he was smart enough to put two and two together and draw his own conclusions.

Thorough history and physical examination were all that were required to help this patient. Coupled with objective evaluation of all the diagnostic test results. Looking at the case with fresh eyes and no preconceived ideas.

Two of the cases I have described demonstrated the danger of tunnel vision. The dog is vomiting, or has abdominal effusion, so let's focus on that body cavity; whereas the problem is actually located in the chest. A thoracic radiograph clinched the deal in both patients. However, there are traps to be avoided here as well. I saw another case, a nine-year-old Labrador cross, who presented with decreased exercise tolerance and "heavy breathing." A chest radiograph was confusing; the trachea appeared distorted as it went through the thoracic inlet and cranial mediastinum. There may have been a soft tissue opacity at the same site. The veterinarian who ultimately referred the case diagnosed a cranial mediastinal mass and – as he had a keen interest in surgery – decided to remove it himself. Unfortunately, the surgery proved negative. On presentation to me, the dog had the characteristic stridor of laryngeal paralysis, and a classic history (except, of course, for the thoracotomy incision). In this case, the referring veterinarian had focused on the thorax as the cause of the respiratory signs and jumped to surgery on the basis of a weird radiograph (the tracheal distortion was probably positional, exacerbated by alteration in the mechanics of ventilation because of upper respiratory obstruction). When we looked at the dog without preconceived ideas, and asked the owners if they had noticed any voice changes, the diagnosis followed quickly.

Sometimes, referral just offers another veterinarian – with the luxury of time – the chance to put all the clues together in one time and place. Something that can be extremely difficult in a busy practice with multiple doctors alternating shifts and duties.

The best outcome is when, having done all of that, we arrive at the same conclusion as the referring vet. I enjoy it when I can say, "I've looked at all the information and I think your vet is spot on. They've done a great job getting us to this point."

Then we, the owners, and the referring vet can collectively make the decision about the next step in diagnosis or treatment. In many cases, the owners will opt to leave the patient with the specialists for treatment, but not always, and only for as long as absolutely necessary.

Harley arrived at Sydney University on a Wednesday morning in the late 1990s, but he had all the hallmarks of a Friday night special. When I left the clinic straight after rounds to give a two-hour lecture on surgery of the lower gastrointestinal tract, I was expecting a very manageable morning of receiving: a smattering of rechecks, a bilateral anal sacculectomy and something that – when booked in late yesterday – was described as "grass seed in the ear."

A low-pressure system dumped over an inch of rain over Sydney just before dawn and, with the veterinary school right at the bottom of Science Road in the lowest part of the campus, the clinic car park became a swamp. The rainwater run-off collected leaves, newspapers, a variety of unidentified and unmentionable objects, and a good deal of mud, all of which was slowly tracked into reception.

I walked into the treatment room at 10:05, expecting a few minutes to discuss the morning's strategy with the students, to be met by a red-faced nurse. Hair was escaping her scrub cap and one of her shirt pockets had been torn adrift.

"I'm glad you're back. Your 12 o'clock's ready for you."

Well, I'm not ready for it, I thought. "They'll have to wait in reception …"

"No, I mean it's in the treatment room and it's ready for you *right now.*"

The treatment room resembled a natural disaster. Storm debris was smeared across the floor, along with an expanding puddle that, judging from the smell, was not water. An instrument tray been overturned, scattering bandages and syringes. Sparkly clean and ready for the day when I left, the room had been completely trashed. As had, it seemed, a number of my students. One sat on a stool with a blood-stained bandage around her hand. Another stood in the corner, figuratively, if not literally, spread against the wall. Two students wrestled with an enormous, filthy creature that emitted an unearthly wail as it tried to burrow its way through the cement floor.

My 12 o'clock appointment: *grass seed in the ear.*

Harley was a 63-kg Bullmastiff who needed three people to prise him from the back seat of the owner's truck when they pulled up in the parking lot. Harley had been behaving like this ever since he was picked up from their local vet late the previous evening.

"Who is the local vet?" I enquired.

"Greenwich Harbour."

Greenwich Harbour was over three hour's drive away. I looked back at Harley; someone had managed to muzzle him and froth was bubbling from either side.

"Did he bite you?" I asked the student with the bandaged hand.

"No, I tore a nail off as we were getting him out of the truck."

"I'll take her down to Anesthesia," said the treatment room nurse. We had appointed one of our anesthetic registrars, with a St. John's Ambulance certificate, as our hospital first aid officer, the first point of contact for any injuries

before they were sent off to the university's Student Health Service, or Royal Prince Alfred Hospital, which was just across the football field at the back of the clinic. She was also the one who chased up the required incident forms after the event. But paperwork was not on my mind as I stared at Harley.

If this truly was a grass seed in the ear, it was the most aggressive I had ever seen. Harley's eyes were flicking violently, his neck was arched to the right, jamming his head into the floor, and his burrowing behavior was a frantic attempt to regain his balance. He was suffering some form of vestibular disease and based on the direction of his nystagmus I doubted it was peripheral.

The horse had already bolted, but I could not curb my curiosity to find out who had opened the stable door. "Who booked this case in?"

"The owners. They said their vet told them he had something in his ear and would need surgery to remove it."

This was clearly an emergency; someone should have seen it last night, and preferably someone closer than 200 kilometers away. I don't know why they settled on the idea of it being a surgical emergency, but nonetheless it landed on my doorstep. I had no idea what was causing Harley's signs, but he urgently needed help, so I gave him some acepromazine for its sedative and antihistamine properties, and hoped that he would settle as we reviewed his record and spoke with his owners.

After taking a history, and performing a thorough physical examination once Harley had quietened down somewhat, it was clear he had a progressive neurological problem. The records from his referring vet were scant, so I phoned for some information.

"Ah," said the vet, "I wondered what they were going to do."

"They seem like a nice couple."

There was a pause. "Really?"

The other side of the story was that Harley had been with the Greenwich Harbour Veterinary Clinic since Monday, with progressively worsening symptoms suggestive of vestibular disease.

The owners, a young couple married less than a month, had no spare money for tests so opted to treat Harley with antibiotics and see whether he improved. At one point the possibility of a migrating foreign body was raised, and it was an attractive option as it was potentially curable. Harley continued to deteriorate with empirical treatment. The owners became progressively more frustrated at Harley's failure to improve, and convinced themselves that Harley had a grass seed, and if it could only be removed surgically he would get better. They arrived at the veterinary hospital the previous night and demanded that Harley be discharged against medical advice, so they could "take him to someone who knows what they're doing." They did not elaborate on their plan, which was to bring him to the university in the mistaken belief we would offer cheap treatment.

A cerebrospinal fluid tap later that day confirmed Harley had granulomatous meningo-encephalitis.

When I delivered the news, they said, "Why couldn't our vet just have told us that?"

I wouldn't be drawn into a discussion of how their vet had tried to raise the possibility, and how they had convinced themselves it must be something else. It wasn't their fault they had no money for diagnostics and treatment, it wasn't their fault they had limited medical knowledge and latched onto the diagnosis that seemed most appealing. All they wanted was to save their dog. Somewhere, though, communication had broken down and the relationship between this couple and the vets who were trying to help them fizzled, and their plans for Harley stopped being objective and considered and became random and reactive.

I prescribed corticosteroids and antihistamines for Harley and within 24 hours he was settled enough to be stretchered back to the truck. He was euthanized at home a week later; I had not been able to cure him, but at least I had been able to make a quick diagnosis.

Many of our referrals are like Harley. The vets or owners know something needs to be done. Maybe they don't know exactly what it is. Maybe they do not agree. Such cases often present for surgery because it seems that medical management has failed and people are running out of options. Our challenge for this style of patient is to work out whether surgery is actually the right option for them and, if not, come up with a suitable alternative. In other cases, the referring veterinarians have got the ball right up to the goal posts, and all we have to do is punt it through.

It was spring in Davis, California. The squirrels were frenzied; chasing one another up and down trees, around the parking lot, and across the cycle paths. The air was full of pollen and everyone was sneezing.

Being April, the students were also looking down the barrel of graduation. That holy grail – such an abstract concept for the last few years – was finally within reach and, as they entered their last few weeks, they were suddenly nervous.

On day 1 of their rotation, I ask students, "What would you like to get from the next two weeks?"

In August, they say, "Anything will be helpful," or "I've forgotten what a uterus looks like."

In December, "I haven't seen a pyometra yet," or "I want to watch a cystotomy."

In April, "I want to learn everything I missed over the last four years."

We had three new cases this morning: a dog with bilateral anal sac disease, another with severe otitis externa, and a third with exercise intolerance and stridor, presumably as a result of laryngeal paralysis. The three students took one each, and spent the morning admitting them into hospital, organizing additional tests, and submitting surgery and anesthetic requests. Because we already had two major cases booked for the following day, we decided to sneak the anal sacculectomy into surgery that afternoon. It was an uncomplicated case; a healthy four-year-old Irish Setter with a long history of anal sac impaction and occasional abscessation. The students were all keen to see this surgery, so they scrambled off to change into scrubs.

I prefer the open approach, so after flushing the anal sacs with dilute chlorhexidine I inserted a surgical probe into the duct and incised onto it to flay open the duct and the sac. Now able to visualize the shiny gray mucosa, I used iris scissors to dissect it from the surrounding tissues, and applied cautery to the twig-like arterial branch that enters the cranial aspect of the sac. I lavaged the resultant wound and reapposed the thin shreds of external anal sphincter that I had divided when the incision was made. The other two students on the rotation appeared just as I placed the last skin suture of 4 0 polypropylene.

They were in shock. "Have you finished already?"

"Sorry, where were you?"

"We had to change, and we thought we better have some lunch before we came in. We didn't know how long it was going to take."

The anesthetist checked her record, "Twenty five minutes."

The students looked crestfallen. I felt a little guilty, but also satisfied.

Later, we Rounded on all three of our morning cases.

"I guess I don't understand," said one student; tentatively, because she did not know how this point would go over in the current company. "Why did the vets refer that anal sac case to us?"

"I was wondering that, too!" said another.

I looked at the student who had received the patient. "What did the owners say?"

"They said their vet didn't seem very confident. They hadn't done many and were concerned about the risk of complications."

"It sounds like they were being honest."

"Yes, but it's such an easy procedure!"

I am cautious about calling any surgery "easy." However, most surgery is straightforward if you break it down into its component parts. You make a skin incision, you identify tissue planes, and do some tissue dissection. You ligate, remove, or implant something. You lavage and then you close. Even open-heart surgery can be broken down into simple steps. If you look at it piecemeal, most vets are capable of performing many if not all of the steps.

"The issue often isn't whether vets are capable of doing it," I said. "Many vets in private practice are excellent surgeons. It's a matter of whether someone is confident they can put it all together from beginning to end. We don't see many complications from bilateral anal sacculectomy, but if we do, they can be major. The most scary is fecal incontinence. And maybe that is less likely if the surgery is done by someone with more experience? And even if the odds don't change, everyone might feel more comfortable that it happened in the hands of a specialist because it is a known complication of the procedure, rather than worry there was a medical error of some sort. If these owners had taken their pet to another veterinary clinic, they might well have had the surgery performed there. Everyone has to work out their own level of comfort with certain things, and that will change as you get more experience."

The students nodded, "That makes sense."

The next day, having confirmed the diagnosis by airway exam, we operated on the dog with laryngeal paralysis. This time, the students who weren't on the case got into the operating room more quickly, but they still missed most of the procedure.

"You've finished *again*!"

"Twenty minutes," said the anesthetist.

"You didn't miss much," said the student holding the retractor. "I couldn't see anything anyway." I glanced at her, and she winked back. I think she was smiling behind the mask but I couldn't be sure. I like it when students demonstrate a sense of humor; it suggests they are outgrowing their existential terror.

For the total ear canal ablation, the students were glued to the dog from the moment it was wheeled into the operating room.

"There are plenty of vets in practice who perform each of those procedures regularly," I said. "Let's talk about how you might make the decision to refer, or to keep it in-house?"

"Lighting," said one student. We had spent a lot of time peering down through a small incision into a dark hole.

"Suction."

"Retraction."

"Surgical equipment."

"Those are all great points," I said. "So let's say your practice has all those things. Including assistants to hold the retractors. I can tell you that the practices who sent the total ear canal ablation and the laryngeal paralysis are both very well equipped."

No quick answer was forthcoming.

I turned to the student on the ear dog. "How confident were you when you looked down Mitch's ear canals that they needed to come out?"

"Not very."

"Exactly. You might think that surgery is the best option, but maybe you want a second opinion. Same thing with laryngeal paralysis. You think that is the cause of the dog's problems but you don't know for sure. And although the surgery might seem straightforward, if you get a complication, or the surgery doesn't work, how is everyone going to feel then?

Sometimes, even here in a specialist teaching hospital we don't know for sure. Sometimes we have to try the surgery and see what happens. That's a big step for someone who doesn't see these cases all the time."

I returned once again to the concept that we visited early in this chapter.

"Diagnosis is key," I said. "Often patients are referred so we can confirm it; either because we have equipment like an endoscope, or because we have the experience. Then there is the matter of surgical and anesthetic expertise. I've seen plenty of patients where the vets and the owners told me they don't care about my surgical expertise, but we have experienced anesthetists."

One vet's exact words (which I will never forget) were "a trained monkey could perform this surgery, but he can't pass gas."

I continued, "In Matty's case [the dog with laryngeal paralysis], we have postoperative monitoring. Her vets made the diagnosis, and they could probably have performed the surgery. But they have nobody on duty overnight."

The students nodded again.

Now we moved to the part of Rounds that I particularly liked. The "what if" discussion.

"What if," I said, "You are working in a practice in …" I struggled for a geographic location that would reek of isolation, "Bear Bottom, Alaska. And Matty came to see you. You were confident that she had laryngeal paralysis and she needed surgery, but referral wasn't an option."

"There are specialists in Alaska."

"Yes, so let's imagine the owners just don't have the money. But they want to save Matty, so they say, 'You do it.'"

"Have I done the surgery before?"

"No. You haven't even seen one before. But the owners are really adamant that you should give it a go. How are you going to prepare yourself?"

"Watch it on YouTube."

"Excellent idea, but there is a lot of sunspot activity and the internet is down in Bear Bottom."

"Read a textbook?"

"Perfect, as long as you have a good surgery text in your practice."

The students got right into the game. "Can I phone a friend?"

"Definitely. But first, how about talking to the other vets in your practice, even if they're not on duty? Find out whether they have seen or done the procedure. Maybe they can come and help you. Two heads are better than one, and they will provide some moral support. And maybe the specialist that you normally refer to would be prepared to talk you through it, if you explain the situation."

"But if there was a lot of sunspot activity, the phones might be down, too. And my colleague might be on vacation in Hawaii."

"Yes, that would be a problem. What could you do then? You would just have to 'go for it,' wouldn't you?"

I had made our scenario so lifelike the students appeared stricken.

"If time allows, how about practicing the surgery first? Maybe you can access cadavers for dissection? Depending on the laws in the part of the world you are working, maybe the local shelters can provide them? I have worked places where we set up a donation system, and some clients were prepared to release their pet's bodies for teaching. There is nothing like looking at the anatomy for real, and not just in a textbook."

In fact, the textbooks can look so different from reality that it's worth spending some time on it in an upcoming chapter.

"And the final thing to consider," I said to the students, "is how you are going to feel if you attempt this surgery you haven't done before, and everything goes wrong?"

There was a collective intake of breath.

"I mean, you've advised the owner that referral would be the best option, and you spoke to them about the potential complications, and they still wanted you to go ahead. And you knew the patient's prognosis was dismal without surgery. So what do you have to lose?"

They waited for the answer.

"You need to think about this very carefully," I advised. "We are all highly motivated and committed people. We expect that if we work hard, and we study and we do everything 'right' we will be successful. We don't deal well with failure. And if you 'give it a go' and it doesn't work,

are you going to blame yourself? Losing the patient on the table would be awful but if it didn't really have a chance without surgery we are usually at peace with that. The owners will probably thank you for trying. But what about the scenario where you operate, and either something goes wrong, or the surgery just doesn't work, and the patient is in a worse state than it was before surgery? And now there is going to be more expense and more suffering than if we hadn't done anything. That is an awful place to be."

"I don't want to be that vet," said one student softly.

"You might feel you have no choice," I said. "And if you take an informed risk and go ahead, I can guarantee you will feel like a miracle worker when it goes well. But make sure, if you do it, that you have prepared in the best way you can, and that at the end of the day, you feel you did the best you could. And also make sure it is your decision to go ahead, and you aren't simply pushed into something you're not comfortable with, because you have to live with the consequences if things don't go according to plan."

5

Courage, Mystery, and Awe

The Intangibles of Being a Veterinary Doctor

Julie M. Meadows

There's so much more to what we do than we can find in the evidence base. We are trained in the specifics of science – how and why the body works, how we can manipulate it with drugs or change it with surgery. Early in our careers the facts consume us, creating a safety net of security and comfort. At some point in every veterinarian's career, though, that safety net stretches – instead of the fine mesh of a strainer, its pores are more like those of a cheap plastic colander, but rather than spaghetti noodles slipping through into the garbage disposal it's our confidence that if we just read the book and follow the steps, everything will be all right. That's when we reach for the intangibles of medical practice – doctoring, courage, mystery, and awe. If we are open to these, we truly become whole practitioners.

It takes some time to develop trust in those intangibles. My professional journey includes 16 years at a private practice in the Central Valley of California, breadbasket to the world, with pet owners ranging from university professors to wealthy ranching families to the immigrants who worked in the fields – and everything in between. In the 1990s and early twenty-first century, these clients had yet to create the demand for specialty veterinary care. As they had for decades, veterinarians dealt with whatever came in the door, referring to practices hours away only for the minority of clients who had the financial resources to reach for secondary care when we had exhausted our repertoire.

In that world, we didn't practice under as focused a microscope as we do now, with less defined "standards of care". If we didn't personally pursue a tentative diagnosis of Cushing's disease, manage our diabetics, and cut our own diaphragmatic hernias, the pet didn't receive care. The human–animal bond is an enduring concept; Pet strollers and "Dogs Being Basic" on Instagram are just visible manifestations of what has existed for centuries – the connection we have with our pets that brings them to us when we cry, yell, cocoon, or play. And rather than see that connection destroyed, veterinarians brought their best to the problems they saw.

The word "doctor" is well defined and historically prestigious. An internet search for the meaning of "doctoring," though, repeatedly ends with words like "falsifying," "adulterating," and other less than illustrious synonyms. In the twenty-first century, doctoring in medical and veterinary schools has come to refer to what we used to call "soft skills"; touchy feely and not based in science. We know, now, that these are teachable skills, distinct from personality or one's Myers–Briggs type. Learning to be a good doctor begins with understanding what we need to know about patients and their families and requires communication, collaboration, and compassion. It is the foundation of relationship-centered care.

Precious, a 10-year-old female intact German Shepherd cross, presented with the constellation of clinical signs you'd expect with a closed

Pitfalls in Veterinary Surgery, First Edition. Edited by Geraldine B. Hunt.
© 2017 John Wiley & Sons, Inc. Published 2017 by John Wiley & Sons, Inc.

pyometra. She belonged to a family who was vacationing on the other side of the country and was presented by her dogsitter. The American College of Veterinary Emergency and Critical Care formed in 1989 but in the late 1990s in California's Central Valley, most vets still cut their own pyos. With fluids, enrofloxacin, and a single injection of Banamine, they generally did alright, although because of the old adage "never let the sun set on a pyo," the diagnosis resulted in a lot of late days for veterinarians. Perhaps because of the absence of her family, Precious had been sick for quite a while by the time I took her to surgery. The most significant finding in her chemistry panel besides mild azotemia was hypoalbuminemia – I gambled that the protein was sequestered in her uterus, rather than being lost from some other cause.

Precious survived the anesthesia and surgery but did not walk or eat the next day; unusual in my experience with post-op pyometras. If ever "a chance to cut is a chance to cure" applied, this is one place where there is no debate. I was about three years into practice ownership and taking advantage of that by letting my parents move their recreational vehicle (RV) to the "back field" of my practice, which had previously been a mixed practice with horse stalls and irrigated pasture. I love my parents, but it was better to have them there than parked in my front yard! My dad, having gotten over his dismay when his daughter did not become a "real doctor," wandered in and out of the hospital regularly and he became attached to Precious and emotionally invested in her recovery. Having a dog's family counting on you to save her is one level of professional pressure; having your dad expecting you to save a patient he's bonded with, after paying for half of your veterinary education, is quite another!

As I worked through Precious' active problems, looking for "fixes," it occurred to me that if I administered plasma I could increase her oncotic pressure, thus protecting her against hemodilution and peripheral edema. Now I know that a single pack of plasma is the proverbial "drop in a bucket," but at the time it seemed a specific therapeutic intervention that might make a difference – and at least it was something I could do. The local emergency clinic, closed but answering their inside telephone line, kept it in stock. My dad willingly popped into my car and drove up for the plasma, returning to sit by Precious' side as she received it. He literally held her hand.

As the day went on and I kept Precious' family updated, they asked to talk to her. So I eventually found myself half lying in her kennel, phone on speaker, watching Precious' ears prick as she heard her kids' voices. Whether it was the benefit of time, the caring spirits reaching for whatever might help, or the sound of childrens' voices, Precious walked out the door three days later. To her family – and my dad – I was a bona fide healer. I suspect mostly I just stayed out of her body's way once her uterus was gone. But I was doctoring, pulling in all the components of care that affect outcome; scientific and otherwise. And Precious and her family were reunited, which is the whole point.

I had been at the practice I would eventually own for two years when a practice even more rural than my own referred a German Shorthaired Pointer, Remi, for diaphragmatic hernia repair. I had joined the two-doctor practice because one of the partners, Tom Browzki, had died of mesothelioma; he had anchored the small animal side while his partner, now my boss, had had a thriving ambulatory practice. Dr. Browzki had developed a reputation as a capable surgeon and outlying practices referred cases beyond their comfort level. Apparently, those outlying practices hadn't gotten the memo that he was gone and I, with my six years of experience, was holding down the fort.

I like cross-stitching and quilting and, in general – if they're not dying – I like diaphragmatic hernias because of the intricate suturing involved, so my stress level entering this surgery was similar to what it would have been for a fat Rottweiler spay.

Until I got in.

Experience had taught me that diaphragmatic hernias were fairly straightforward: identify the rent in the diaphragm, bring the displaced organs back into the abdomen, align the torn muscles of the diaphragmatic crura, and place closely spaced simple interrupted sutures to close the gaps. The hardest part was problem-solving how to re-attach the diaphragm if it was completely torn off the body wall. This, however, was not a recent trauma patient – Remi had been hit by a car weeks before – and when I tried to pull the cranial liver lobes and right kidney back into the abdomen, they wouldn't budge. It was as if they were glued to the pleura. It took me a few minutes to think through the problem, identifying that the organs were no doubt, at this point, fibrosing to their new locations. Centimeter by centimeter, I blindly, digitally, broke down the adhesions holding them in place, aware that the wrong angle of a finger would bore a hole into a mushy parenchyma and cause hemorrhage that would likely, in a place with no readily accessible blood donors, lead to death by exsanguination, or pneumothorax if that parenchyma happened to be lung. Twenty-two years later, I still remember wishing Remi would die – I felt like I was in a nightmare from which I couldn't escape. But she didn't. Debbie, the technician who stood at her head and manually pressed the rebreathing bag for those interminable hours, had cheered me on through complicated spays and she did the same for this dog. Eventually, the organs were back where they belonged, the torn diaphragm repaired, the air removed from the pleural space, and the abdomen closed. No liver hemorrhage, no pneumothorax, no re-expansion pulmonary edema. Remi recovered uneventfully and went home; no doubt to chase another car.

Those of you who've been through this know how my neck ached, how much I craved an icy Dr. Pepper, and how much I just wanted to go home. For those who are just beginning your careers, and asking questions from this book, know that many of the answers are already inside you; you just have to find them. You either decide to make a difference, knowing the depth of your education and remembering that, ultimately, outside of the anesthetic challenges, things like diaphragmatic hernias are exercises in suturing and critical thinking, both of which are fundamental skills possessed by all good veterinarians, or you step back and send the patient further along the referral chain.

I encourage you to make a calculated decision when the time is right and step up to the plate – be courageous! Our society has some clients with unlimited financial resources, and many more with finite limits on what they can spend for pet care. The former have access to the highest realms of veterinary care, in tertiary referral centers throughout the country. But there is a larger group of clients who love their animals just as dearly, and for whom that level of care, or even referral to your local emergency clinic, will be beyond their economic realm. If surgical intervention is required for survival or quality of life, and if you recognize in your heart, that you know what to do but you've just never done it before, think about whether you can be truthful with your client regarding your level of experience and offer the appropriate intervention. Only by doing can we grow, and only by doing can we save lives.

In 1991, Rachel Remen, a pediatric oncologist by training, designed the Healer's Art curriculum to provide for a personal, "in-depth exploration of the time honored values of service, healing, relationship, reverence for life and compassionate care".[1] Originally offered to first and second year medical students, it was opened to veterinary students in 2012. The curriculum consists of a series of large and small group sessions on individual themes. One of the themes is "mystery and awe"; while each student of healing is encouraged to speak to what these mean for themselves, the foundation of the theme is being open to and feeling safe with events in medicine that are beyond science.

No doubt any battle-scarred care provider would be able to summon an experience of the mystery and awe inherent in medicine. Mine

---

1 http://www.rachelremen.com/learn/medical-education-work/the-healers-art/

was with an aged Sheltie, Prince, who presented with vomiting and diarrhea. His family, tightly bound to him, was traveling around the country in an RV and far from their home base and home veterinarian. Not knowing me from Adam exacerbated their worry. It also made things more challenging for me, as my entire way of being a veterinarian is based on having a relationship with my clients upon which trust is established. Over the course of Prince's hospitalization, I found an intestinal mass and, in non-metropolitan California, referral to a board-certified surgeon was not automatic. I took him to surgery.

I found the mass at the ileocecocolic junction. The thing about intestinal anastomoses is, intimidating though they might be to those of us who have never done them or who don't do them frequently, the principles of the procedure are straightforward: cut the intestinal segments at the correct angle to maintain their blood supply and be sure your incision doesn't leak intestinal contents after you've sutured the segments back together.

So, knowing the couple was sitting in my lobby, I proceeded to remove the mass. Only once I was ready to anastomose did the luminal size difference between the ileum and colon register with me – my pieces didn't "fit" together. To me that's the biggest difference between theory and experience. We can practice self-directed "book" learning all we want but eventually we all come across something we didn't anticipate or that didn't go the way we expected it to. Where we go from there reflects back on that question about courage.

In a world of relationships, I've tried to cultivate good ones with the specialists to whom I refer. Those individuals' responsiveness when I reach out to them is the prime determinant of whether I will refer to them again. Most surgeons have dedicated technicians with whom they work who have the ability to immediately access their doctor. Respecting those technicians' role and access makes life easier. Happily, for Prince, Paul Canfield (my second favorite surgeon of all time), came to the phone to help

in my crisis. It turned out he had no magic solution – there rarely is in medicine and surgery. My best option was to maximize the diameter of the ileal segment by cutting more obliquely than normal and then anastomosing it with as much of the distal segment's lumen as possible. That left a blind pouch at the antimesenteric border of the colonic segment, and, it seemed to me, a single spot of extreme suture line vulnerability. I proceeded, but there was definitely a right angle where it didn't seem to me that the incision was locked up tight, even though the repair passed the leak test.

As I spoke to Prince's family post-op, I gave the standard speech about the potential for dehiscence and voiced my concern about that single spot, telling them we had about four days to wait and we'd know he was out of the woods when he pooped. As they settled their RV onto the grounds (I had begun to think I should open a combination RV park/concierge veterinary care!), I sat with closed eyes in front of Prince's kennel and envisioned God's index finger plugging that triangle of vulnerability. This was long before a sister-in-law introduced me to the concept of affirmation. At the time, she had a picture of her dream house posted where she saw it regularly – she had faith that house would materialize for her family. With a misunderstanding of the true definition of affirmation, I felt like if I could just draw upon spiritual energy and channel it to a place of true need, Prince's incision would heal. (Little did I know I was supposed to be programming my subconscious, not God's will.) But over the next few days, in concert with traditional medical care, I kept my faith that God would keep that finger lightly resting on the incision. Images of ET – the Extraterrestrial's glowing digit also floated through my mind, suggesting that I was hedging my bets by channeling more than one celestial being. Days later, when Prince pooped a normal stool, we were all jubilant. Prince's family drove on to whatever came next, sending me a Valentine's Day card from the road months later. I deferred their thanks, though – accepting with awe the power of healing, in all of its dimensions.

6

Placed on Earth to Test Us

The Not-So-Humble Spay

Catherine F. Le Bars

The term operating theater has always seemed an appropriate name for a room that sees more tension, tears, and sweaty relief than any other room in a veterinary hospital.

The phrase came into use during the eighteenth century, when students and other interested parties would seat themselves about a table and watch the local sawbones ply his trade, with the aid of recycled strands of thread, the sweepings of cotton mills, and monstrous instruments steeped in brandy. In those days, the experience of watching a conscious being subjected to the blade proved as entertaining and marginally more educational than Nero's gladiatorial games of Ancient Rome. The advent of general anesthesia dampened the screams and broadened the audience but in no way lessened the high drama found in such medical amphitheaters.

Clients often tell me "they'd love to have been a vet but couldn't stand the suffering." I am not sure whether they refer to our patients or me but I suspect that I have acquired more gray hairs in the theater than I would care to calculate. Since many of these occasions have seen me elbow deep within a family pet's abdomen, it is in that vast red cavity of glistening tubes and very large vessels I intend to spend the rest of this chapter.

I shall focus on the humble ovario-hysterectomy. One of my favorite procedures, which is fortunate really, since I have been obliged to remove more ovaries from dogs, cats, and pocket pets over the past 28 years than I have had cooked dinners.

Vets I have known fall readily into two categories when it comes to bitch spays: those who accept and even relish the challenge and those who do not. The latter category can be further divided into those who approach each spay as a test of fortitude and indomitable spirit, and those who employ an inventive array of tactics to remove their initials from the operating list on spay day.

So what is it about this routine procedure that inspires equal measures of satisfaction and fear? Well, first it is an elective procedure and therefore there is everything to lose if events go ill and, second, there is nothing routine about it.

We promote National Desexing Month each July, when we offer half-priced neutering to all and sundry in our local area. A procedure, already heavily subsidized by the profession, for 31 days costs less than a color and perm and, perhaps unsurprisingly, that's when the really "fun" ones come in. The six-year-old Doberman with tits down to her creaky knees, the Staffy with roughly the shape and mobility of a beach ball, followed closely by my personal favorite, the aged Kelpie that may or may not have had a season this year but almost certainly has a dubious vulval discharge that has prompted the farmer to finally fork out a few bob on having it "dissected."

These are the ones that sweat me back into shape and have me wishing I had followed my

Pitfalls in Veterinary Surgery, First Edition. Edited by Geraldine B. Hunt.
© 2017 John Wiley & Sons, Inc. Published 2017 by John Wiley & Sons, Inc.

mother's advice and become a florist. But they are also the patients that have honed my skills and forced me to become increasingly creative in the theater.

I once spayed a hamster brought into the hospital by a young lady who had found it behind the bins at McDonald's. It was a quiet day and I was fascinated by this tiny creature resembling a water bomb balloon with paws. Plus, our rather dour practice manager, Sharon, had unaccountably taken a fancy to the hamster and given it a name. Without knowing what to expect, we anaesthetized Big Mac and removed an ovarian cyst the size of a golf ball. In the absence of obvious metastases, I removed the other gonad and the rather sweet-tempered, now slimline rodent lived a further six months with Sharon.

My advice to inexperienced colleagues on the subject of spays can be applied to most procedures and summed up accordingly: respect the first principles of surgery.

Clip enough fur to allow yourself sufficient access, with room to extend the incision if required. Be decisive with your incisions, rather than worry the soft tissues apart with a myriad of tiny tugs and tears. Treat tissues kindly and they will reward you by not dehiscing. Additionally, there is also a very good chance the animal won't feel obliged to remove its own sutures. Select your suture material with care and, most importantly of all, learn to tie a square knot!

And be patient. Most ovaries will see the light if you apply gentle traction for long enough. When you do encounter a fatty monstrosity anchored to a distant spine in a slippery sea of oily omentum, don't be afraid to extend the incision or request an extra pair of hands. It is a simple fact that some spays were placed on Earth to test us.

Oh, and don't forget to tell the owners what you are planning to do. Over the years, I have honed a pre-operative speech I present to my clients with all the fervor of Henry V addressing his men at Agincourt.

The speech serves two purposes. It advises owners that the ovario-hysterectomy is not a routine procedure and it covers my back for

those, thankfully rare, times when events don't run according to plan.

I ask that they consider a pre-operative blood test to ensure that their healthy young pets are indeed as healthy as they believe and to obtain a baseline should future testing be indicated. It is surprising what those tests throw up from time to time even the most boisterous of youngsters.

Next, I run through the basics of the procedure itself because it is surprising how many clients don't actually understand what they are giving us permission to do. This was brought home to me last year when a client returned her Poodle for a "routine" post-op check. The conversation went something like this …

"And how is Diamond today? She looks pretty lively."

There came a pregnant pause, accompanied by a reproachful glare.

"She is *beyond* trauma!"

The owner proceeded to tell me that the tiny black poodle dancing about the room on her hind legs was in a terrible state as a result of having lost her womb. The owner would never have given her consent had she known we planned to remove the ovaries AND womb. Apparently, the loss had tapped into a similar trauma suffered in her previous life, also as a poodle. Diamond's survival during the past few days had apparently little to do with my surgical skills and all to do with the pendulum, crystals, and aromatic salves the owner had diligently applied.

It all seemed a little unfair and more than a bit crazy but then it struck me that this client had a point. I should have discussed the details of the procedure prior to surgery and not assumed an underpinning knowledge.

On the subject of underpinning knowledge, I must mention that our clients are occasionally guilty of the same assumption. To protect us and our patients, our Hospital has a pre-neutering checklist (honed over the years) that we ask the clients to sign. One of the questions reads, "Has your pet eaten anything unusual in the past few days?" This question has prompted a few surprising answers, including at least two clients who thought their puppies had eaten a "bit of rat bait" last week but hadn't thought to mention it at the time of booking the appointment.

And then there is the list of additional procedures such as deciduous teeth, hernias, and dew claws. There are few things more aggravating than noticing the reducible umbilical hernia during the surgical prep while simultaneously discovering that the "contact" number provided by the client was not actually a means of reaching them on that particular day.

Beware of emergency spays. These are the ones squeezed in at the last minute by a kindly receptionist because the owner must have it done the following day. They often arrange to drop the pet off at first light even though it is the first time we have seen it. The reason for such urgency is usually not apparent on the booking note but immediately surfaces once the bitch has been admitted and the owner has departed for work. The contact number is of course linked to either a mobile that has run out of charge or a landline missing one digit. I can almost guarantee that these bitches will either be in raging pro-oestrus or about to push out a sackful of puppies.

Finally, a quick word about the humble pyometra – one of the many reasons I have an ultrasound machine in the surgery. Point out the pus to the client and you will rarely hear them debate the necessity of an emergency ovario-hysterectomy.

I prefer to reach the pyos before they turn green and burst but on the occasions I have arrived too late, the bitches do remarkably well with the right care. As a new graduate I was horrified when my boss back then, an elderly chap with an encyclopedic knowledge of the world and an explosive temper, advised me to simply sew the linea alba loosely and leave the poison to drain.

I followed his directions cautiously and rather than eventrate on the floor of her pen, this particular bitch leaked for a handful of days then proceeded to heal as uneventfully as the thousands of dogs I have since sutured dutifully in line with the dictates of my surgical lectures from university days.

It is beyond the scope of this chapter to discuss the many reasons we enter an abdomen; however, I would like to say just two things … expect the unexpected and be prepared. Because how ever many radiographs we may have taken, blood tests we have run, or scans we have performed, it is surprising what lurks within.

7

"Oops!"

Not a Good Word to Hear During Surgery

In terms of their behavior under stress, surgeons tend toward two extremes. The classic caricature is of the "instrument thrower"; hurling curses and curettes to equally devastating effect. The "distressed" surgeon becomes frantic and rough, but tends to reduce communication to a bare minimum, leaving their assistants to try (often unsuccessfully) to work out what they need next. Other surgeons become icy calm, often to the point that others in the room have no idea that anything is out of the ordinary.

Early in my career, faced with a difficult situation, I began to shake. I was calm in most other respects, but my hands gave me away, and no matter how much I tried to stop them, they tremored like my own emotional seismograph. It might not have mattered had I been doing a dog spay in my own practice, but when it happened during an open-heart procedure surrounded by captivated surgery students, it was a problem. I read about how to control shaking during surgery, and became progressively more interested in the phenomenon as I advanced from resident, to junior Faculty, to Head of Surgery. As time went on, I also discovered that my presence alone was sufficient to set my own students quaking.

"Stabilize your wrist on a solid object," I told them. "Sometimes the only convenient platform might actually be your assistant. But do ask their permission first! In the absence of a willing assistant, be careful not to lean too hard on the patient's chest.

"Remember to breathe, and work on other techniques for resolving anxiety. Think through the things that you fear about this surgery, and how you might deal with complications if they arise. Take time out to reflect on what you are doing and ground yourself. Having a plan can reduce a lot of stress."

My own tremors resolved with time; probably as I became more experienced and developed confidence that should there be a mishap in surgery, I could probably deal with it. But although I controlled most external manifestations of stress, I never completely stopped shaking on the inside.

Some people shake as a result of caffeine, medication, or a condition known as "essential tremor," so it is worth getting a medical opinion if simple solutions don't help. It should be possible for most people to control their tremor enough to perform the routine surgeries common in veterinary practice, but it may be that shaking does preclude some people from doing advanced surgery. In my experience, though, there are a lot of things for a student or young veterinarian to try before they make that career call.

After spending two years in small animal practice in Canberra, I followed my dream of becoming an academic by enrolling in a PhD. I had become captivated by electrocardiography in the final year of vet school, and wanted to learn everything possible about electrical activation of the heart, so persuaded the Cardiology Department at a large medical teaching hospital in Sydney to take on a veterinarian for their translational research program. They didn't use the word "translational" back in those days, but

Pitfalls in Veterinary Surgery, First Edition. Edited by Geraldine B. Hunt.
© 2017 John Wiley & Sons, Inc. Published 2017 by John Wiley & Sons, Inc.

as we were testing concepts in the animal lab that were then applied upstairs to their human patients – often within weeks – it seems a good description.

Laurence, the cardiac surgeon I worked with on our experimental patients was of the unflappable variety: always polite, always calm, and very good at what he did. I was standing across the table from him, using an Allison lung retractor to its best effect while he cannulated the aortic root of research dog No. 16, when he demonstrated his state of relaxation by commencing to whistle "Every Breath you Take" by The Police.

"Uh, oh!" It was the anesthetist.

It turned out this particular surgeon's response to stress was to whistle, and he only ever whistled when things were heading south.

It came as a surprise to me – but no great shock to the people who knew Laurence well – when the aorta tore open and the chest began to fill with blood.

With no pause in his whistling, Laurence stuck his finger in the hole … *every move you make* … then searched around on the instrument table for a vascular clamp … *every vow you take …*

Had I been a better assistant, I would have predicted this need, located the Satinsky immediately and passed it to him, but I was so horrified by the amount of blood – and my gut-dropping certainty that this particular patient was beyond help – that I was temporarily incapable of doing anything useful.

Laurence had whistled his way through to the final verse by the time he had the side-clamp on the aorta, I had suctioned the blood from the thorax, and he was performing a neat continuous closure of the vessel using 5-0 polypropylene on a tiny taper needle. The anesthetist showed great restraint in withholding shock quantities of intravenous fluids until the bleeding was actually under control, and within five minutes of Laurence commencing to whistle, the patient was stable again and we were able to move to Plan B. Laurence had not even broken into a sweat.

I had; sweating and hand-shaking seemed to go together, and although I did overcome the hand-shaking issue, I never got on top of the hyperhidrosis.

Once Laurence stopped whistling, everybody relaxed.

"The worst sort of bleeding," he said to the room in general, "is bleeding you can hear."

He then informed me that things weren't really under control until you could slow the bleeding to a "dull roar."

A handful of years later, after I finished my PhD and started my surgery residency, I watched one of my own patients bleed out on the table during repair of a patent ductus arteriosus (PDA). We clamped, suctioned, and desperately tried to find the leak in order to seal it. Our anesthetist poured in crystalloids, whole blood, and colloids, but they all ended up in the suction canister and we called it a day when the dog went into ventricular fibrillation for the third time. A totally miserable situation for everyone, and one that I wanted to avoid experiencing again.

Dr. Chris Bellenger, my great mentor and supervisor at the time, debriefed me on this episode, discussing all aspects of the surgery and anesthesia to see whether we might have done anything differently. It made me reflect on Laurence's handling of surgical crises. How did he manage to save his patient, whereas we lost ours?

Trying not to panic is a good first step, but rather hard and not really an end point. Having a plan helps me to avoid panic, because I can shift straight into the plan without having to think too hard. The value in knowing exactly what my first steps will be is one of the many things I learned from life outside veterinary science.

Like most Australians who grow up in coastal towns, I have always loved the ocean: as a kid I spent my weekends and holidays on the water, in the water, and under the water. After years of sailing and generally messing around in boats, I bought an ocean kayak and started to explore Sydney Harbour. On clear mornings I would launch from Balmoral (one of the harbor beaches) and paddle out towards Sydney Heads to watch the sun rise. I taught myself how to ride the wake of the Manly ferry, stabilize myself in the backwash of the Pacific swell hitting Middle Head, and do whatever I needed to avoid tipping over. When I decided to extend myself and sign up for a 100-kilometer kayak race down the Hawkesbury River, however, I decided it was time to take a lesson (Figure 7.1). My two-hour private session focused on how to survive a capsize, and took place on a crisp winter morning. The sun was out, but the water was a bracing 13 °C (55 °F). I was dressed in thermal kayaking skins, wet weather gear, and life jacket. I was secured into the kayak with a spray skirt fit tightly around the cockpit rim.

"The first thing," said the instructor, "is to feel what it's like to roll your boat."

This seemed rather basic; I was an ocean swimmer and knew all about waves and cold water.

"When you flip," said the instructor, "you will want to follow these steps:

1) Run your hands up either side of the kayak and hit the hull firmly. The banging noise alerts other kayakers that you have turned over.

2) Slide your hands back up to the cockpit rim, then work your fingers forward to feel the tab on the spray skirt.

3) Pull the tab firmly down and to the side. Don't pull the tab directly upwards as you might hit yourself in the face.

4) Let yourself slide passively out of the cockpit.

5) Surface next to the kayak and immediately grab hold of it."

Hardly brain surgery, but he made me run through the drill two or three times while I was upright, until we were both happy that I remembered the steps.

"I am going to flip you over on the count of three," he said. "One, two …"

Dark water closed over my head and rushed up my nose.

Shit! I thought, realizing that I was upside down and trapped. *I'm about to drown!*

I couldn't have predicted that feeling of shock considering I knew exactly what was about to happen and precisely when. My brain shut down and my immediate urge was to wrench the spray skirt off and kick my legs hard to force my way out of the cockpit. It took a concentrated effort to get myself under control and remember that

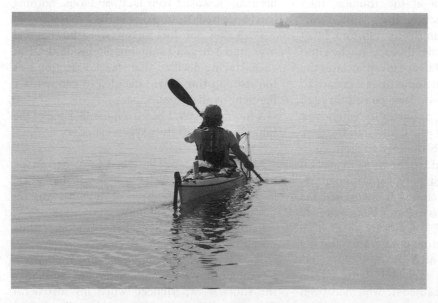

Figure 7.1 Kayaking can teach you a lot about how to cope with the unexpected during surgery. Courtesy of J. Bourn.

all I had to do right now was execute the first step I had just learned.

Run your hands up either side of the kayak and hit the hull firmly.

After that, everything unfolded smoothly, and within a few more seconds I was bobbing next to my kayak, holding onto the sideline, and positioning myself for the T-rescue that we were due to practice next.

Fast forward to Mocha, a fat Yorkshire Terrier who presented for the classic goose-honking cough of collapsing trachea. The cross-section of Mocha's trachea resembled a crescent moon, which underwent a total eclipse on expiratory radiographs, thus explaining the dog's inability to walk more than a few steps without collapsing. In a situation where intraluminal stents were not widely available, Mocha's combination of cervical and thoracic tracheal collapse imparted a poor prognosis, but Mocha's owners really wanted to try, so I made a ventral midline incision from the hyoid apparatus to the manubrium sternum, and commenced placing rings cut laboriously from a syringe case amidst a fair degree of foul language. The cervical trachea was easily accessible, but the more I widened it, the worse the trachea at the thoracic inlet looked. With a little traction, and a limited sternotomy incision through the manubrium, I was able to advance the cranial thoracic trachea into the surgical site. I should have given up after the first couple of rings, but sometimes it is hard to know in surgery when you have passed through that glorious portal of opportunity where you are making positive progress, and into the dark corridor of progressively diminishing returns.

"Just about done," I said to the room in general as I positioned the last polypropylene suture. But before I started to close, I thought, *Just one more ring; with some dissection I think I can get just a little further back.*

I snatched the retractors back from Sam, my puzzled student assistant.

"Just a bit further," I explained, ignoring the rolling eyes of my anesthetist, who had been through this play act before.

I gently slid the atraumatic forceps down either side of the trachea to check how free it was. The next most caudal ring was tantalizingly close; almost completely dissected apart from a small fibrous band on the right-hand side. I held out my hand, "Lahey's, please."

Sam was a good student and had anticipated my request; he placed the instrument promptly in the palm of my hand using his most excellent technique. I inserted the instrument into the dissection plane beside the trachea, only to notice that the right-angled forceps I had been expecting was actually a pair of Metzenbaum scissors.

"Yikes!" I whipped the scissors away from the trachea before I cut anything.

Sam sounded as if he were being strangled, "You didn't want Metzie's?"

"No problem," I said lightly, "my fault. Be very careful when you're asking for instruments," I said to the rest of the watching students. "Make sure you speak clearly, and always check that the instrument you are given is the right one."

Sam was a tall blond surfer dude from SoCal. Usually the class clown, at this moment he looked about to burst into tears. Such is the effect that we surgeons have on people. I touched his arm, "It wasn't your fault, and look, nothing bad happened! Now, pass me the Lahey's."

The Lahey bile duct forceps were duly handed over, and I began tunneling alongside the trachea. Having decided that sharp dissection was too risky in this area, I decided to gently tease the tight band of tissue apart.

A moment later, I heard a noise like one of the tubes bursting off the oxygen cylinder.

"What ...?"

As that single word emerged, I watched an arc of blood erupt from the base of Mocha's neck, leap the drape at the head of the table, and hit the anesthesia resident between the eyes.

In that moment, I recalled Laurence telling me about bleeding you can *hear.*

The shock of hearing and seeing my patient bleeding out from a major artery was similar to the shock I experienced when my instructor flipped my kayak over. You can't really prepare yourself for it, and when you're upside down and drowning you shift to survival mode.

I plunged my finger into the tunnel from which the blood had erupted.

"Okay," I said, as much to settle my thoughts as for anything else, for this was bleeding you could also *feel*. "That's a pretty big leak."

I had the rapt attention of everyone in the room. No chatting about plans for the weekend, or sneaking out the smart phone to check the latest postings on Instagram. I had them in the palm of my hand; or would have, had I dared move it from the base of Mocha's neck.

The anesthesia resident was wiping blood from her glasses and the anesthetic monitor. I could have told her what the blood pressure was, though.

"Okay," I said again. "Sam, pick up the Pool sucker and start suctioning blood from around my hand."

Sam had gone sheet white.

Please don't pass out right now! I thought.

To Sam's credit, though, he controlled his shaking well enough to get the nozzle in the general vicinity of the wound.

"With your other hand, get some laparotomy pads down here," I said. "Now, I need an artery clamp."

Sam fumbled through a tangle of blood-encrusted instruments on the table and produced a tiny mosquito forcep.

"Bigger," I said, adjusting my finger to occlude the jet of blood still thrumming into my palm.

Sam extricated a Carmalt clamp about the same length as the dog.

I reached across with my free hand and grabbed a Kelly off the table.

"I would normally say that digital pressure is enough to control most bleeding," I said. "But not in this case." My shocked audience looked on in silence.

The anesthetist had cleaned the monitor sufficiently to tell me that Mocha's blood pressure was dropping.

I channeled Laurence, the cardiac surgeon. "Bleeding you can hear is never a good thing," I mumbled, partly to calm my nerves.

I was thinking, *Oh God, have I made a hole in the aorta? How am I going to get a clamp on it? How close am I to the heart? What about the trachea? What about the vagus nerves? What am I going to tell the owner?*

I don't usually recommend placing clamps blindly when trying to control bleeding; you never know what else is going to end up in the jaws, but I broke that rule now. I slid the tip of the clamp as close to my finger as possible, trying to include minimal tissue. I clamped something, and had Sam lavage and suction the wound dry before I removed my finger. I also had laparotomy pads to pack into the wound if the bleeding continued.

Wonderfully, and to an audible sigh from the onlookers, there were no more gushers as I withdrew my hand from Mocha's neck.

"Okay," I said again, noting my audience had increased to an even dozen in response to the primal magnetism of a crisis in a veterinary teaching hospital.

"It seems the bleeding has stopped, but let's check and see whether this clamp is across anything important."

I turned to the anesthetic resident; now being advised by her Faculty who was standing a sensible distance from the splash zone. A quick check of systems showed that the airway was still patent and the dorsal pedal arterial catheter was still reading pressure, suggesting I had not cross-clamped either the trachea or the aorta. *Phew!*

I prised the suction nozzle from Sam's clenched fingers and replaced it with a malleable retractor.

"Breathe," I told him, and, although I didn't quite believe it, "Everything's under control."

Carefully, with gentle flushing and suctioning, I investigated the surgical wound around the site of the forceps and found I had clamped the right common carotid artery, close to where it arises from the brachiocephalic. Not wanting to risk the manipulation required to pass a suture, I called for hemoclips, and placed three across the site at a variety of angles, checking after each one that the brachiocephalic pulse and caudal arterial pressure did not drop. Then I applied Gelfoam, and further packed the region with gauze to encourage hemostasis while we tidied our instrument table, cleaned our hands and the instruments we would need for closing, and generally got ourselves back together.

"It wasn't your fault," I told Sam again. "The vessel tore because I shredded it with the right-angles."

Torrential bleeding was potentially not the only mishap we were dealing with, though.

"Chances are, I've also clamped the vagosympathetic trunk." I slipped into teaching mode, "What signs are we likely to see in recovery if I've done that?"

Sam gave me a classic "deer in the headlights" look. "Diarrhea?"

His emotional state following the horrible drama of his first surgical case was evidently not compatible with a rational discussion of the autonomic nerves of the neck. Either that or he was alerting me to his own physiological urge.

Struggling for a response that would not add to Sam's misery, I said, "Possibly. Let's think about it some more while we finish the surgery."

"I take it you won't be placing any more rings?" the anesthetist said drily.

We surgeons can't help ourselves; just one more ring, just a little tighter on the suture, just a little more dissection. In our defense, we are trying to get the best result for the patient. I keep pushing further because I have a sneaking concern that I haven't yet done enough to make a difference to this particular dog or cat. I haven't closed the hernia tightly enough, removed enough disk material from around the spinal cord, attenuated the portosystemic shunt sufficiently, explored the abscess thoroughly enough.

And once I'm on a roll, few of my colleagues are brave or confident enough to try to stop me. So I have to recognize this situation when it occurs, and look at it objectively. *Am I really making a difference now, or am I doing more harm than good?* But giving up when you're not sure whether you have completed the job you set out to do is so hard! In this particular instance, it was left to my patient to tell me that

enough was enough; which he did in no uncertain terms.

"While we close up and get Mocha into recovery," I told Sam, "let's work out what complications to look for, and what we need to warn the owner about."

With escalating paranoia, I was thinking, *I didn't mention any risks of nerve damage other than laryngeal paralysis, and I certainly didn't discuss damage to the great vessels of the chest. And who knows whether the surgery is actually going to help anyway?*

So, how can we synthesize these collective experiences into an approach for an "oops" moment like torrential arterial bleeding?

First, as I experienced during my controlled kayak roll in the relative safety of Sydney Harbour, it is going to be a shock, regardless of how prepared you are. And if it is a shock to you, imagine how it's going to feel to your assistant (if you have one), or the vet tech who is urgently summoned to scrub in, the work experience student, or some other bystander?

Second, we all react differently to shock and stress: some withdraw, some yell, some whistle. What we should do is recognize what our personal response is, and learn to keep communicating regardless. Laurence was an excellent and effective surgeon, but the fact that we had to wait for him to begin whistling to know that things were getting curly was not satisfactory. I have to force myself to explain what is happening when I get stressed. I would far rather put my head down and work on the solution than bother explaining myself to other people, but that is wrong. It is far better to verbalize our thoughts than keep them to ourselves.

Maybe not the *I wish I was anywhere except inside this dog!* or *What the hell do I do next?* type of thought, but certainly the *I am having trouble with visualization and am going to shift the retractors and dissect a little further to find out where I am* variety.

I know that I get terse under stress; not very polite and rather "grabby" with the instruments. I don't remember throwing anything across the room, but niceties go out the window. I have taken to apologizing to my assistants ahead of time when I think we might be heading into that territory. I explain how I am likely to behave and reassure them that they will all have an important and valued role, no matter how it might seem at the time.

It is also important – albeit hard – to listen to your colleagues when you are struggling, for they may have very good suggestions and ideas to contribute.

There are also things we can do before trouble strikes, if only we think about them.

How differently might our experience with Mocha played out had I taken the time to run quickly through the anatomy of the area with Sam before surgery, and the process should we encounter an unexpected problem? If we had agreed on the best instrument for Sam to pass in the event of hemorrhage, made sure we had one on the table, and kept it clean and separate from the other instruments so we could get it quickly? In Chapter 9 we will talk about "How to be a fast surgeon," and a situation like Mocha's is a certainly good time to be fast.

When we lost our PDA patient to hemorrhage, Professor Chris Bellenger and I discussed the things we might do to prevent such a problem in the future, and we developed a "fire drill" in which we ran through the scenario with our assistants, worked out where everyone's fingers and hands should be, and made sure we had instruments and everyone in the team knew what the steps would be if and when it happened again. It did happen again, in four patients over the next few years, and we saved the three for whom we followed the drill.[1]

Fortunately, intraoperative bleeding is usually not the type that we can hear, and we have time to react. We may perforate a major vein and not even know it if the central venous pressure is low; but the next time the positive pressure ventilator cycles, the venous pressure peaks and a tsunami of blood floods the surgical site. Venous pressure is thankfully low and, unless you have made a huge hole, venous bleeding will often resolve with digital pressure. If it doesn't, one or two cruciate sutures of a fine monofilament suture (4-0 or 5-0 polypropylene on a small taper needle) positioned directly across the bleeding site might be sufficient to stem the tide.

More commonly, we drop an ovarian pedicle, or see oozing from the broad ligament or splenectomy site. You can apply pressure with your finger, as I did in Mocha's case, but a wad of moistened gauze swabs is preferable as long as you do a thorough sponge count before you close.

Remember to apply pressure for long enough. Five minutes is good, 10 minutes is better; but that's an awfully long time in surgery and you can only measure it accurately with a stopwatch or clock.

While you wait, calculate the patient's circulating blood volume and try to work out how much has been lost. What volume does a soaked surgical sponge hold?[2] How much is in the suction canister? By the time you have done all this, the bleeding has probably settled to a "dull roar," and you will have realized that you have some time to correct things before your patient bleeds out.

When you are ready, peel the laparotomy pads or sponges away one at a time, progressively exposing the surrounding tissues, which you can inspect for bleeding. Eventually, you will lift the sponge directly off the bleeding site and, hopefully, the leak will have stopped. Resist the temptation to lavage your organizing blood clot away. Pack the site again with surgical sponges and leave it for a few minutes while you clean up your surgical table, or check the rest of the abdomen.

A word about clamping: if the vessel is large enough to worry you, there is probably another

1 Hunt GB, Simpson DJ, Beck JA, *et al.* Intraoperative hemorrhage during patent ductus arteriosus ligation in dogs. *Veterinary Surgery* 2001; 30: 58–63.

2 5–18.3 mL. Zeltzman P, Downes MO. Surgical sponges in small animal surgery. *Compendium of Small Animal Practice* 2011; June: E1–E8.

important structure nearby, be it a nerve or something else. Blind clamping is not usually a good idea. Mocha woke up with Horner's syndrome that never completely resolved, and I've seen at least a handful of patients with hydronephrosis as a result of ligatures applied when a bleeding uterine vessel slipped down beside the cervix, and the hemostat picked up the ureter as well as the artery. Repeated clamping and suctioning also leads to greater blood loss and can interfere with local mechanisms for hemostasis. My approach: clamp if I can see the bleeding point, otherwise go straight to pressure and packing.

If bleeding continues after pressure and packing, it can be helpful to flood the site with warm saline, suctioning and reflooding the area until the fluid is clear enough to see through. Bleeding points appear as wisps of red "smoke" where the blood spirals gently to the surface. This is useful for body cavities but also for large soft tissue wounds where you can make a well using the surrounding skin.

Remember also that the blood might be coming from another site. I once spent over an hour trying to find the source of blood that kept pooling in an abdomen only to discover that it was trickling down from the laparotomy incision. The cranial abdominal vessels on either side of the xiphoid are notorious for this, and can be hard to find within the falciform fat pads.

Of course, hemorrhage is only one of the unexpected events that occur during surgery. Contamination is another, and is best dealt with by avoidance, or copious lavage and suction. The complications that scare us most, though, tend towards two categories: cutting – or ligating – something we shouldn't.

When you cut a large artery, as I learned repeatedly, you usually know straight away. But some errors are not apparent immediately, and these are the most insidious, as the delay in detecting and characterizing them impedes us from mitigating the damage or treating the consequences.

Bennett was a nine-year-old Foxhound with a large bilateral perineal hernia. Bennett's diagnosis was straightforward and his condition stable: his bladder was not retroflexed and apart from being miserable because of chronic constipation, he was in good shape for anesthesia and surgery. I helped the resident and the surgical repairs went smoothly. Bennett had underwhelming coccygeus muscles but we tacked everything together and the end result was solid. We took out his anal purse string suture, removed the tampon from his anus, did a rectal examination, and congratulated ourselves on a good job.

Bennett was a wimp in recovery. He woke up screaming and it took multiple doses of opiate along with acepromazine and a shot of phenobarbital to settle him down, rendering him unable to walk back to his ward at the end of the day. He spent a restless, uncomfortable night, so first thing the next morning we decided to get him out of his cage and check him more thoroughly. When we asked him to get up, he screamed. This seemed far more serious than routine postoperative pain, even for a rather "dramatic" patient.

I have learned that if a patient displays an exaggerated and unexpected pain response, it is usually not because they are being temperamental, but because they are exquisitely painful and quite possibly from a cause unrelated to the surgical wound itself. I had one patient who was tachycardic and vocalized all night after an exploratory celiotomy; five days later we discovered the third degree burn on her back. Another patient screamed when we tried to move her following a foxtail exploration; she had a cervical disk prolapse.

As Bennett walked from his cage, there was clearly something wrong with one back leg; he knuckled and his hock had dropped. He didn't favor it, as with a sprain or fracture; he just couldn't use it properly.

I have seen large dogs that were recumbent for a long time show temporary signs of peripheral neuropathy (neuropraxia) for a few moments after getting up; similar to the situation when our leg "goes to sleep." I have also seen dogs with underlying spinal disease (chronic disk protrusion or wobbler syndrome) become worse immediately after anesthesia and surgery. And don't forget the potential effect of an epidural on limb function within the first few hours after surgery. But, in Bennett's case, the combination of intractable pain and peripheral neuropathy were highly suggestive of a surgical complication. I had never seen this particular complication before, but I must have read about it, because it sprang straight into my mind.

"Sciatic nerve damage," I told the students.

When I diagnose nerve damage in a patient postoperatively, I immediately wonder how I could have been so stupid as to cut the nerve. At what point in the surgery did my attention wander? Which of those fibrous attachments did I not check carefully enough before dividing?

Once I've stopped blaming myself, I start to blame the patient. It is a great temptation to implicate "inflammation" or "hematoma" because that is something that can resolve with time (and without forcing us to that very uncomfortable step of *going back in)*. And if you have cut a nerve, is there much point to *going back in* anyway?

I worked through this dilemma out loud for the benefit of the students and resident. The chances were we either cut the sciatic nerve during surgery (unlikely because of the pain Bennett was showing) or we skewered it with one or more sutures while trying to get purchase in the coccygeus muscles. If the sciatic was merely entrapped, and the suture had not completely crushed it, then the sooner we released the suture, the sooner we could relieve Bennett's pain, and hopefully allow the nerve to recover.

"We need to go back in," I said.

The resident went to call Bennett's owner, and the surgical technician went to the operating theaters to submit an emergency anesthesia request, leaving the rest of us to ponder what "going back in" actually meant in this case. The natural thought would be to open the surgical site (at least we knew which side was affected), and remove the sutures likely to be causing the problem. The trouble with that approach was

that Bennett would still have his perineal hernia, and we would again be faced with the difficulty of finding substantial enough muscle to perform a repair, with the added complication of now-traumatized muscle and a desire to take shallow bites so as to avoid a second insult on the sciatic nerve.

"We could do a superficial gluteal flap," one of the students offered.

"Or use the semitendinosus," said another. They were a very good group of students that week.

"You know," I said, "I think it's unlikely that we placed multiple sutures around the nerve. Possible, but I suspect there is just one. If we could find that single suture, we could remove it without taking the whole repair apart."

Surgeons have to think three-dimensionally. Use our knowledge of anatomy to devise surgical approaches for situations that do not fit the textbook. In this case, the answer was to explore the sciatic nerve at the location where it was most likely to be affected; just cranial to the sacrotuberous ligament. I had not approached that region before (at least not deliberately) so we found a copy of Miller's *Anatomy of the Dog* (dog-eared, tattered, some pages falling out and others spotted with blood) and got to work. That is how a textbook should look, in my opinion: much handled and – if not loved – at least well-used (Figure 7.2).

Having researched the anatomy and chosen a lateral surgical approach to the pelvic canal that should expose the sciatic nerve and sacrotuberous ligament, we anesthetized Bennett and prepped him for a complete perineal hernia revision along with superficial gluteal flap in the event it was required. Then we did our lateral approach and as soon as we got to the target area, saw a single, blue polydioxanone suture pinching the caudal half of the sciatic nerve. Another suture was very close to the nerve, but not actually impinging on it. Snipping the offending suture was a simple matter and Bennett's leg gave a satisfying twitch, which gave us hope that the affected neurons could still transmit. We debated whether to do anything further and decided to simply close the

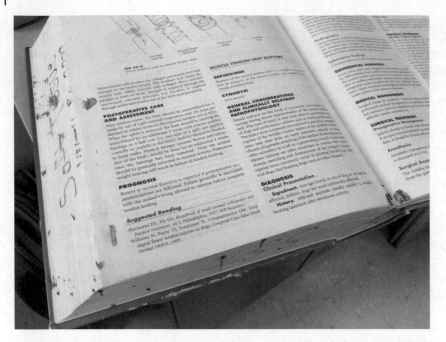

Figure 7.2 A well-loved surgical textbook.

wound, recheck the perineal hernia repair (it still felt solid on rectal examination), and hope for the best.

This time, Bennett woke up like a normal patient following perineal hernia repair; no screaming, no need for industrial doses of sedatives and analgesics. When he walked from his cage, he still had some nerve impairment, but we persuaded ourselves that it seemed better than before, and indeed it largely resolved over the course of about two weeks, during which time we put his hock in a brace and he wore a protective boot on his foot.

Bennett was lucky that we detected his problem in time to do something about it, although in retrospect we could have made the diagnosis a lot earlier, and saved him a night of pain, and some residual dysfunction.

No matter how much experience you have, you will encounter the unexpected during surgery. Everybody has mishaps, but I think we show our experience and competence in the way we respond once they have happened. If we think ahead, and make contingency plans that we can follow at a moment's notice, then we can get ourselves out of trouble and also be a safety net for those around us. And, as we will discuss shortly, when we are flying on the surgical trapeze, a safety net is a really important thing.

8

Learning the Hard Way

Student, Resident, Teacher

All this talk of surgical mishaps naturally brings me to the troublesome patient I introduced in Chapter 1. As I already mentioned, I grew up on the Northern Beaches of Sydney. It was an idyllic place in the 1960s and 1970s: yellow beaches strung like pearls along a rocky coastline, huge inland waterways, large areas of bushland, flocks of brightly colored parrots, and very little traffic. Our home on the peninsula between Pittwater and the Pacific Ocean was at the end of a two-lane, winding road over an hour's drive from the city center. In winter, the place was almost deserted. On warm weekends in spring and summer, day-trippers flocked to the beaches, but not in sufficient numbers to warrant a set of traffic lights.

My pre-school sat amongst a stand of eucalyptus trees that harbored the last koala colony of the Northern Beaches. We heard the males bellow during mating season; a mechanical cacophony at odds with their cuddly appearance. One morning we were ushered quickly inside as a muscular old buck strolled through our yard; his claws were enormous.

With all its bushland, Avalon was also home to a healthy population of Eastern bandicoots and, with them, the paralysis tick, *Ixodes holocyclus*. For those of you who have never practiced on the east coast of Australia, *Ixodes holocyclus* is a seriously nasty creature. Not only do the adult ticks cause an often-fatal paralysis, but huge numbers of nymphs infest the local vegetation in late summer and autumn. We call them grass ticks and they can shower you in the hundreds; miniscule and undetected until delayed hypersensitivity ignites a constellation of intensely itchy spots.

My first experience with our local veterinarian was when our golden Labrador, Honey, fell sick one wet November morning. She uncharacteristically refused her breakfast, vomited shortly afterwards, and commenced to stagger around the kitchen, her hind end swaying from one side to another. She had previously been diagnosed with hip dysplasia but this was different. We rushed her to the local vet who was, coincidentally, situated right next to my preschool in a three-room fibro garage. We used to play in the shadow of its crumbling walls so I was dismayed when I recently discovered that the building material we called "fibro" is more appropriately termed asbestos cement sheet.

Dr. Lewis discovered an engorged adult tick embedded in Honey's antitragus (I had to look this up – it is the floppy fold just caudal to the ear canal), diagnosed tick paralysis, and administered antiserum. Up to 40% of dogs die in years when the ticks are particularly venomous, but Honey was one of the lucky ones and she was returned to us two days later (Figure 8.1).

Dr. Lewis fascinated me. He was in late middle age, thickening about the waist but still possessing a fine head of hair. He had cheeks that might one day become jowls and reminded me of Fred Flintstone. He traveled overseas regularly and impressed me enormously by not only having *met* Stephen Ettinger but being in regular communication with him. At the time, Sydney seemed so remote from North America, and Avalon Beach was so remote from Sydney, that

Pitfalls in Veterinary Surgery, First Edition. Edited by Geraldine B. Hunt.
© 2017 John Wiley & Sons, Inc. Published 2017 by John Wiley & Sons, Inc.

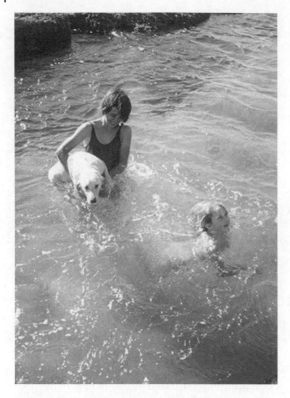

Figure 8.1 Embryonic Dr. Hunt and her sister, Kate, teaching Honey how to swim.

Dr. Lewis actually knowing the American who wrote the major textbook on veterinary internal medicine was akin to him being on speaking terms with the man in the moon. I came to think of the unprepossessing fibro garage as a portal to the rest of the world, so when I reached my third year of veterinary school and needed to arrange some external practical experience, I knew where I must go.

Thus, I found myself in charge of an enraged rainbow lorikeet.

Screech! Screech!

These colorful psittacines are captivatingly playful, chatty, and just plain entertaining as long as nobody upsets them. When upset, they emit a noise completely incommensurate with their small body size, which resembles two pieces of polystyrene rubbing together.

Screech! SCREECH!

The noise was accompanied by frantic fluttering and scratching along the asbestos cement wall, which brought Dr. Lewis from his consulting room. He threw a dishcloth over the bird, which immediately went quiet. Thus neutralized, the lorikeet allowed him to cradle it in one hand and examine the spindly leg that jutted at an unnatural angle from its breast feathers. A Good Samaritan had found the bird tangled in a net placed over his kumquat tree. At some point during its frantic and exceptionally noisy imprisonment, the bird had fractured its tibiotarsus.

It was a quiet day in the practice and I can only imagine that Dr. Lewis was trying to keep me occupied, because he suggested we anesthetize the bird so I could apply a splint to its leg. We placed the lorikeet in a plastic box and gassed it down with halothane. Then we inserted its head through the hole in a plastic glove taped over a cat mask, in order to maintain gaesous anesthesia. I was to straighten the limb, cut a matchstick to size, and fix the splint in place with a tiny strip of adhesive.

It might have been a good plan, had we not been using a Stephens anesthetic machine. Everything went smoothly until the moment I started to secure the splint around the bird's leg. My patient, who had been seemingly unconscious, its chest making tiny excursions that moved virtually no air across the vaporizer, suddenly came alive. It pulled its head from the mask, screeched, and flew sideways across the operating table, trailing a jess of Elastoplast.

While I stood – paralysed – Dr. Lewis displayed surprising alacrity by flipping his trusty dishcloth like a matador's cape and scooping the bird from midair.

"Be quick!" he instructed me.

I freed the strip of bandage from the bird's tail feathers, finished wrapping it around the splint, and gently pressed it back onto itself. We then released the lorikeet –voicing his polystyrene serenade – into a birdcage.

"You can look after him at home until its time to remove the splint," said Dr. Lewis charitably.

We called the bird Laurie – of course – and he quickly became a family favorite. He would chatter constantly to himself, or anyone else within earshot, and loved to eat fruit; so we poked pieces of watermelon and banana through the bars of the birdcage. Every day, I changed the newspaper and refilled his birdseed and water, and he tolerated this calmly as long as I did not get too close. On the first occasion my probing hand violated his personal space I discovered that, in addition to his remarkable set of lungs, he had a very sharp beak.

He sparked great interest amongst the rest of the family, being my first proper veterinary patient. My grandparents came to visit, and he greeted them with a musical if not melodious monologue. He seemed no worse the wear for my surgical interventions and hopped about happily on one leg while the other recuperated within its matchstick and Elastoplast splint. Our Labrador, Honey, also wiggled in on the act. She was very close to my grandparents having for many years – without our knowledge – abandoned our house when we left for school and work and trundled the kilometer and a half to their place; where she took her morning snack of Vegemite sandwiches. Sadly, the gentle exercise proved no match for her calorie consumption and in later years she came to resemble an ottoman coffee table.

Delighting in the attention, Laurie pranced and chortled and hopped while my closest family members marveled at his good spirits and wondered when the splint would be removed.

Dr. Lewis and I determined that if a dog's leg healed in six weeks, a bird's leg would probably heal in two, so the day for splint removal came quickly. I was now an old hand at taming lorikeets, so I quickly captured Laurie with a dishcloth. I then asked the closest of my fascinated entourage to hold him while I extricated the broken leg and carefully cut away the Elastoplast with nail scissors. I gently flexed and extended the exposed leg and it didn't flop around. So far so good.

"The bones appear to have achieved clinical union," I informed my family, who looked suitably impressed at my facility with this scientific terminology.

I retrieved custody of Laurie from my father and pushed the bird – still wrapped in his tea towel – into his cage. I drew the fabric away and quickly removed both it and my hand before he could nail me with his beak. He gave one quick squawk and retreated to his perch.

I leaned forward – aware of my gathered family's bated breath – to better visualize my first surgical masterpiece.

"Is it supposed to look like that?" my mother asked.

I felt like crying. Laurie balanced on his perch with one foot, as usual. He held his other foot with claws tightly clenched – and pointing towards his tail. In setting Laurie's leg I had achieved almost 180° of external rotation. I had not yet learned the correct medical terminology for this orthopedic complication but my younger sister, Kate, knew exactly how to describe it.

"It's on backwards!"

The incident became firmly engraved in our family history and – in their eyes at least – a defining moment in my veterinary career.

Available evidence suggested Laurie was far less bothered by his malunion than I was. And although the original plan had been to release him as soon as he was healed, he was so popular with my family that everyone felt he might be better off living with us permanently. So Laurie became a fully fledged member of our household. My best friend from school had a budgerigar who was so tame they let him out of his cage each evening. He would perch on the back of the sofa in the television room and amuse himself for hours by talking to a spot on the wall. Laurie became so tame that after a week we took pity on his incarceration and decided he too should be allowed the freedom of the house. When I opened the cage door he hopped out, tilted his head to one side, and flew straight through the living room window. Not even a "thank you" screech as he went.

I expect he did alright. Suburban Sydney was richly inhabited by people trained to feed the squabbling beggars that flocked daily to their balconies. They gave the breeding pairs names such as Romeo and Juliet, Bonnie and Clyde, and Antony and Cleopatra. We liked to imagine that some backyard bird feeder might one day be visited by a peg-legged Laurie and – perchance – even a Lorraine.

Despite the embarrassment of Laurie's leg-setting, it became clear during the following years that I was meant to be a surgeon.

In my last year of vet school, captivated by the patterns and logic of myocardial activation, I set my sights on veterinary cardiology, until my research degree taught me that I preferred the instant gratification of correcting things surgically to the delayed and uncertain exercise of palliating them with medication.

But as I walked into the Sydney University Veterinary Clinic on the first day of my residency, I was overcome by doubt.

Would I be able to do this? Could I learn what was needed? Why should people trust me with their pet? How long before I made a mistake and proved that I wasn't as competent as people thought?

It was ameliorated somewhat by the fact that I had already been in practice for three years, and spent another three years doing experimental surgery for my PhD. In some ways I felt extremely competent and experienced; in others I was a complete novice, and that was very unsettling. As I looked through the operating room windows while one of the senior residents repaired a humeral fracture I couldn't wait to join them, but my heart pounded.

Fortunately, I had an easy start. The first case I ever logged was a 15-year-old Poodle called Burman, with a pigmented mandibular mass. In months to come I would learn that pigmented oral masses are often malignant melanomas, and that they should be biopsied and staged prior to excision, but for reasons not recorded my supervisor and I decided to simply remove it. My log shows it to be a benign melanoma, with no recurrence after two months. My residency was off to an auspicious start.

It didn't take long for the bubble to burst. Like all veterinary Faculty, worldwide – as far as I have seen – our supervisors were pulled in many directions. It was Monday morning and I was admitting dogs for the weekly spay clinic we ran with the students. My Faculty was 40 miles away at the rural campus, teaching more advanced surgical procedures to the final year students, when Bosco presented to Internal Medicine. Bosco was a red Australian Cattle Dog, about three years old, who had been acquired from a friend and recently developed abdominal enlargement. He dragged behind the owner as they entered the waiting room; head down and chest heaving. A quick physical exam revealed his abdomen to be full of fluid and his mucous membranes blue–gray. A chest X-ray from the referring vet showed his chest to be full of something that was not air. Further scrutiny turned up linear gas shadows that looked suspiciously like loops of bowel. A focused ultrasound showed stomach and liver lobes cranial to the diaphragm.

Having just spent three years doing experimental open-heart surgery, I knew my way around the chest. Repairing a diaphragmatic hernia did not seem much of a stretch, so I bumped the spays and took Bosco to surgery.

I made a stab incision in the linea alba and a flood of serosanguinous fluid erupted from his abdomen, causing me and the students to jump. Even when you know it isn't blood, the sight of something gushing from your patient under high pressure is disturbing. We scrambled to get a suction probe into the abdomen before the flood began shorting out electrical equipment. The nozzle sank straight into the falciform ligament, and Bosco's peritoneal effusion soaked the drapes and Bair Hugger™ before cascading down my leg and over my shoe. I gathered myself enough to extend the incision and evacuate the remaining fluid in a more elegant fashion. I even had the presence of mind to collect a sample for analysis.

Bosco did have a diaphragmatic hernia; apparently chronic, based on the retracted and fibrotic diaphragmatic remnants. His organs slid easily back into the abdomen, with the exception of his liver. His quadrate lobe was reflected and torsed, and adherent to his pericardium. While I suspect most new residents might be intimidated by handling the heart within their first week, I was in my element. I stripped off the adhesions and returned the dark-looking quadrate lobe, with its attendant gallbladder, to its rightful location.

The diaphragm repair was tight, because of the retraction on either side of the rent, but it came together and Bosco's linea alba closed easily enough. We placed a thoracic drain to evacuate air slowly from the chest over 12 hours to avoid re-expansion pulmonary edema. The students and I considered it a job well done, and Bosco was wheeled to recovery as we forged on with our afternoon of spays.

My Faculty supervisor, thinking he had left me safely occupied watching the students break suspensory ligaments and tie square knots, did not check in that evening. The next morning we skipped rounds and moved straight into a morning of receiving elective surgical cases, so we didn't discuss Bosco then either.

Bosco recovered uneventfully from surgery. He was breathing almost normally, and seemed brighter on his morning walk. I did feel a little guilty about taking a case to surgery without any discussion with my supervisor, but we had been sure of the diagnosis and I was confident in my abilities in the thorax. Bosco refused breakfast, but he seemed stable and, because I was moving on to other surgical cases, I removed his chest drain and transferred him back to Internal Medicine, with a view to sending him home the next day.

My surgical supervisor and I spent the rest of the week evaluating and operating on a candy-store selection of orthopedic cases. I logged a L7-S1 laminectomy, transverse humeral fracture, intercondylar fracture, atlantoaxial instability, femoral neck fracture, and shoulder osteochondritis dissecans.

Bosco remained in hospital. The night after the surgery, he still had not eaten and seemed dull. He had some abdominal fluid on palpation, but nothing spectacular, and we decided it was probably left over from surgery. The following morning, his abdomen was clearly enlarged. His breathing was okay, though; his heart was readily audible and his cardiac impulse palpable. I breathed a sigh of relief; at least the hernia repair was still intact!

That seemed little comfort, though, as Bosco's condition continued to deteriorate and his abdomen swelled. His bill passed the estimate we had given before surgery and Bosco's owner had just about run out of money. With Bosco in no fit condition to go home, and his abdominal distention worsening, we faced an escalating crisis.

Nowadays, I tell every resident coming onto my service that we are part of a team: if they find themselves with a problem that they can't resolve quickly, ask for help.

It hadn't occurred to me to ask for help with Bosco at the beginning. His diagnosis seemed obvious and the surgical solution was uncomplicated. In reality, I was also struggling with the transition from being a practitioner – and a PhD trained in advanced cardiac surgery – to a resident, and I wanted to prove that I was a capable surgeon in other respects as well. Had I asked for help with Bosco, I probably would have been advised to either wait until my supervisor was available, or hand the case over to a more experienced resident.

But I did not, and now things were going south, and the only person I felt I could turn to was myself. Which was not a lot of help, as I was becoming progressively more nervous about the situation. I ran through a list of reasons that Bosco might have ongoing peritoneal effusion, and none of them were very good. I was particularly concerned about the possibility of a surgical complication. Had I sutured the diaphragm too tightly and occluded the caudal vena cava? Had I created a splenic torsion? Or had I (*please, no*) left a surgical sponge in the abdomen?

The Internal Medicine resident and I conferred, and we spoke with Bosco's owner. In the days before computerized medical record keeping and billing, it was easy for us to make an executive decision to run some further tests free of charge. We would keep Bosco under the radar until we worked out what was happening and where to go from here. An abdominal radiograph showed fluid but (*thank goodness*) no radio-opaque sponge marker. Biochemistry revealed hypoproteinemia, hypocholesterolemia, low blood urea nitrogen, and hyperbilirubinemia. It seemed Bosco was going into liver failure.

It was a glum procession of surgery and medicine residents, followed by a distended, unhappy dog, who walked out to the lawn that evening. The situation did not improve when we returned to the building to find the hospital superintendent and the Head of Surgery watching us.

I gulped in anticipation of "What are you doing with this dog?" or "Why are you treating patients in secret?" or "Come to my office immediately."

Instead, my supervisor commented calmly, "He doesn't look like he's doing very well."

By the next morning, Bosco was head-pressing, pacing, and generally disorientated with presumed hepatic encephalopathy. In consultation with the owner, and our respective Faculty, we decided to euthanize Bosco. He was sent to pathology and a sense of impending doom settled over me as I waited for the necropsy results and the inevitable summons to account for my unprofessional behavior.

Bosco was shown to have hepatic cirrhosis, presumably as a result of chronic quadrate lobe torsion and compromised blood supply to his liver. The fluid in his abdomen was a pure transudate and had we sampled it during our postoperative work up we could have ruled out things like retained surgical gauze and Budd–Chiari syndrome secondary to the hernia repair, as they would have led to a higher-protein fluid, similar to that which was seen during the original surgery. We finally concluded that Bosco's clinical signs escalated when his liver lobe torsed, the portal hypertension resulting in a florid abdominal effusion that overflowed to the thorax through the diaphragmatic defect, prompting his owners to take him to the vet.

I was hugely relieved: Bosco's surgery might not have cured him, but at least I hadn't done anything seriously wrong.

I didn't get called to the Head of Surgery's office, which I find amazing because if one of my own residents behaved in a similar way tomorrow I would take it up with them immediately. But although it seemed I got off lightly, the real result was that I was left to learn this particular lesson in a far more brutal way.

Although I absolved myself of responsibility for Bosco's outcome, and persuaded myself that I had acted fairly professionally under the circumstances (you can draw your own conclusions), I realized I should keep my head down and defer to my supervisor during the coming weeks. I was on an orthopedics rotation, and my logbook shows a succession of extracapsular cruciate repairs, arthrotomies, and fractures. Although I knew a lot about the heart and great vessels, I knew very little about orthopedics, and I soaked up knowledge like a piece of Gelfoam.

Telly was a six-month-old German Shepherd with premature closure of his distal radial growth plate. During a month of limping after he tripped over his human-brother's Tonka truck and fell down the stairs, his right front leg began showing obvious signs of an angular deformity. This was a condition I remembered from vet school, and I enjoyed working through it: the obvious cause and effect, the orderly process of analyzing radiographs, measuring angles and performing the osteotomy to correct the defect, then applying an external fixateur.

A couple of weeks later my supervisor was again teaching off campus when I was summoned to the treatment room by one of our primary care clinicians.

"Take a look at this leg."

Tramp was a 10-week-old Bullterrier cross whose breeder had noticed him knuckling over on his left front carpus. He didn't have much angular deviation, but there was clearly a growth abnormality and he was favoring that leg.

"The owner's been giving him cage rest but it's getting worse."

I had learned a lot from our recent case of radial growth plate closure and felt I had a good grasp of what was needed to diagnose and correct Tramp's problem. I ran through it all with the clinician and we costed it up.

"That's expensive for a 10-week-old pup."

"Or we could amputate."

"Seems extreme. I doubt they would come at that."

We knew that severe arthritis would set in if the problem was not corrected, and maybe even if we did attempt surgery. So it didn't seem there were too many options.

"I'll go talk to him," Tramp's clinician said, and walked out to reception.

Half an hour later, my supervisor returned from his surgery lab and, mindful of the Bosco incident, I ran the details of this new case past him.

"Oh, that's just a ligament problem," he said offhandedly. We see it in young, rapidly growing dogs that have exercise restriction. Has he been kept in a cage?"

"Yes."

"Tell them to let him out of the cage and it will get better."

I had never heard of such a thing. I certainly hadn't read any reports about it.

"Has this been published?"

"No, but anyone who sees a lot of orthopedics knows about it."

I felt like an idiot. "I'll go tell his clinician."

"I think you're too late."

I followed my supervisor's gaze across the room. Tramp's clinician was injecting a dose of Lethabarb. The puppy sank to the table; his eyes open, tongue protruding between tiny deciduous teeth, strangely knobbly front legs splayed apart.

"They didn't have any money for the surgery and they didn't want him to suffer," his clinician explained.

My supervisor looked at me, and my heart sank. This beautiful young puppy was dead because of the advice I had given. It had seemed so straightforward based on my previous experience. I had no idea about this dynamic contracture of young, growing dogs.

I realized then that I might know a lot about some very limited topics, but there was so much I didn't know, and I couldn't learn it all from the literature. We all worry about making mistakes during surgery, but my misdiagnosis and its resultant cost estimate resulted in the owners choosing to end Tramp's life, when he actually had a condition that would have resolved spontaneously if he was just allowed to do what young puppies do so well: run around and play.

I didn't need to be hauled in front of the service chief, or the hospital director. I fled the building with a heavy heart. I wasn't cut out to be a surgery resident. I was an idiot and I had killed this puppy with my ignorance.

A referee for a prospective surgery resident once told me, "He doesn't know nearly as much as he thinks he does."

That described me perfectly. It was the first time I seriously considered giving up my dream of becoming a surgeon, and that is not a feeling you forget.

The catch with not knowing what you don't know is that it is very hard to avoid mistakes like the one I made with Tramp. The condition of flexural deformity of the carpus was written up three years later[1] and hopefully all veterinarians now recognize it, but perhaps not? And what other syndromes are out there that become complicated or even lethal because we just don't understand them yet? Which is why I say to all my residents, over and over, *make it a habit to ask your supervisors for their opinion.* Even if you don't think you need it. Because you never know what you don't know, and it may save someone's life.

---

1 Vaughan LC. Flexural deformity of the carpus in puppies. *Journal of Small Animal Practice* 1992; 33: 381–384.

9

"But I Don't Want to Look Stupid ..."

How to Let Others Help You

We cross a number of watersheds in our careers, moving from the role of student to instructor, and back again. As we accumulate qualifications, people naturally look to us for more and more of the answers. It is critical while we mature as veterinary professionals to develop confidence in our knowledge and our ability, and accept that we have a right, and also an obligation, to provide advice and undertake treatment. On the flip side, we are always learning; we will never know everything there is to know and, even after decades of experience, our knowledge will not be identical to someone else's. We can always benefit from discussing our cases with other people.

It is hard to ask for advice, though, especially when you are the doctor (or the resident, or the specialist, or the professor). Asking for advice seems akin to asking for help, and if you have to ask someone else for assistance, what sort of impression does that give? Do you hear a confident, experienced professional pleading for help?

How did it feel the last time one of your colleagues asked you for advice? Did it feel like desperation because they didn't know what to do? Did it feel like they respected you and were genuinely interested in your views? Did it feel like they genuinely wanted to explore every avenue in order to get the best outcome for their patient? When they asked, did you feel the major focus was on them, on you, or on the animal in their care?

I used to hate asking for help; it made me feel weak and vulnerable, and suggested that I couldn't find my own solution to a problem. I also loathed it when someone else asked me for advice and then failed to take it. I wondered why they even bothered asking. But I responded even more poorly to someone who didn't ask advice when I knew I had information to offer, and then proceeded to do something badly. As the situation deteriorated, and they become more flustered and stressed, it became harder and harder to find a way to help.

Some of the greatest learning moments of my residency, and my years as a junior Faculty, were related to the asking for and giving of advice.

There is an old adage; never ask a question to which you do not know the answer. This seems ludicrous to me; surely you should be asking in case someone else does know the answer.

Try to focus on the outcome (finding the answer) rather than on yourself (trying not to appear stupid). You will look a lot more stupid if you act without knowing an answer that your colleagues have at their fingertips, or if you wait until things are so out of control that it literally is a desperate call for help.

And be generous when someone else asks honestly for help. There is no law set in stone; we don't have to ask. We can sew up a wound, send a patient home, or even euthanize it if we want to cover up our failures. It takes courage to expose ourselves when things are not going well; to listen honestly to other people's opinions, and be prepared to change our treatment plans. We have to make it about our patient, and not about us.

In addition to reminding me that I did not know as much as I thought, the other thing my

Pitfalls in Veterinary Surgery, First Edition. Edited by Geraldine B. Hunt.
© 2017 John Wiley & Sons, Inc. Published 2017 by John Wiley & Sons, Inc.

experience with Tramp (the growing puppy with the ligament problem from Chapter 8) taught me was to search always for the simplest explanations and solutions to a problem. As our knowledge grows and access to technology improves, we are able to offer progressively more and more complicated services. When I described Tramp in surgery rounds, over 20 years after his death, I asked the students what their recommendations would be. They chose plain radiography, ultrasound, CT, and a nutritional consult. This is a textbook answer: educated, scientific, thoughtful; but if we lose our perspective we risk complicating the simple. Maybe this is a phenomenon of veterinary teaching hospitals, but I suspect from chatting with others that it happens everywhere. Tramp's owner would never have agreed to radiographs, let alone CT – and those tests would not have yielded a definitive diagnosis, anyway – so the thing most likely to have helped him was advice from an experienced, yet practical, veterinary "elder."

I worked with a number of visiting surgeons during my residency. These people had either just finished a residency or were on study leave from other schools. I was therefore exposed to many different ideas and ways of doing things. We were introduced to the latest concepts from the UK and USA, some of which we took on board, others that we dismissed as fads. Being Australian, I preferred to make up my own mind about things, rather than accept them simply because "everyone" was doing them overseas. In fact, to an Australian, the term "this is how we do it at …" is simply an invitation to prove there is a better way.

One of our visitors, Rachel, had come straight from a residency in the Midwest USA. She was a lovely person to work with; willowy thin with long, glossy hair and a quiet demeanor at odds with our preconceived ideas about Americans. We worked together on a number of cases, including an elbow arthrodesis, total anal resection for a dog with perianal fistulae (thank goodness they found a way to treat that disease medically!), and a comminuted femoral fracture

that took over eight hours and remains the longest surgery I have ever scrubbed into. Eight hours is too long, especially if you are the assistant. We entered the operating room at 10 o'clock in the morning and emerged after everyone had gone home for the night. In the final stages of the surgery, I dropped a pair of needle holders into the trash and was so mentally and physically tired that I reached down to pick them up before I caught myself.

Later that week, the other surgery resident admitted a major orthopedic case and requested Rachel's help. I was left with Missy, an 11-year-old Afghan Hound with chronic ulcerative otitis externa. Previously a docile, affectionate dog, Missy had become withdrawn and lethargic, and aggressive when anyone approached her ear. Her owners were at their wits' end.

"If you can't do anything to help her, we'll have to put her down," they said tearfully.

Missy's ear was severely inflamed and ulcerated, but did not have the hyperplastic changes usually associated with end-stage otitis. Nevertheless, medical management was not helping, and although the ear was still anatomically functional, a total ear canal ablation (TECA) seemed the only feasible way of restoring quality of life for Missy and her owners.

I ran the case past Rachel, who agreed. She would not be available for the surgery, but Missy's owners had made it clear that she needed either immediate surgery, or euthanasia.

"You have good soft tissue skills," said Rachel. "You'll be able to handle it."

I was flattered by this expression of confidence, and went back to the owners.

"We can do the surgery tomorrow."

"That's wonderful!"

Then they asked, almost as an afterthought, "How many of these have you done?"

I hesitated. I personally had never done one. I had never even seen one.

"Oh, we do them regularly," I said lightly. I had, without thinking, slipped into a lifelong habit of using the royal "we." Usually reserved for religious leaders or sovereigns such as the Queen of England, the royal "we" allows us to take refuge beneath a mantle of assumed corporate knowledge. I knew Rachel, and my other supervisors had done these cases. The senior residents had certainly logged them. If "we" did such cases regularly, then surely "I" could also do them.

I did run into trouble with the royal "we" once. A vet referred a Doberman with a cervical spinal lesion and I sent the owners away until the following week because the image intensifier was being repaired. When the owners reported back to the vet, she phoned me to voice her strong displeasure.

"These people drove for three hours to the university for surgery, and all you did was order some blood tests?"

"We thought we should test for von Willebrand's and hypothyroidism."

"Who's 'we'?" she demanded.

I was taken aback: nobody had called me on that before, "Well, I mean, 'I' did."

"So you didn't discuss it with anyone else?"

Again, I struggled to respond, "Yes, we always talk about our cases."

There was little I could do to appease her, and our conversation finished on a very awkward note. The honest truth was that I hadn't really discussed it with anyone; there seemed little point as I couldn't do any imaging at that time anyway. But in using the term "we" I had subconsciously persuaded myself that I was representing my whole surgery service, and that was not true. The veterinarian's formal complaint led me to the hospital director's office to explain myself; an unpleasant but no doubt character-building incident.

Fortunately, Missy's owners were appeased by my use of the collective, and listened as I ran through the potential complications. We all agreed that this was Missy's last chance, and surgery was set for the following day.

I read the textbook the night before, and practiced the surgery in my head as I tried to sleep.

Missy proved an excellent case for my first TECA. Being a sighthound, she was lean and, because her ear disease was characterized by mucosal ulceration, there was little inflammation

external to the ear canal and the cartilage remained thin and pliant.

"It's not as if she's a Cocker Spaniel," said Rachel, as she disappeared into the orthopedic operating room. "They have rocks attached to their skulls. But call me if you need any help."

I didn't need to call her; the surgery went smoothly and methodically. I cauterized the myriad small bleeders, teased apart the fibrous attachments to the ear canal, held my breath as I curetted mucosa from the osseous ear canal, and sweated as I nibbled bone off the lateral tympanic bulla.

"The dorsolateral aspect of the bulla is the most critical," Rachel had warned me. "That's where people tend to leave mucosa, which leads to a draining sinus."

Two and three quarter hours later, Missy's ear canal was on the surgery table, and I was lavaging a sparkling clean tympanic bulla. I placed a Penrose drain, closed the wound, and waited on tenterhooks until Missy recovered enough to demonstrate a brisk palpebral reflex.

I had done it! All on my own! Even more rewarding, Missy seemed comfortable and relaxed virtually from the time she went back to her run. When they took her home, Missy's owners said she had regained her personality. Even with the pain of surgery, removing the chronic focus of her discomfort had been enough to make life worth living again.

I did not look back from that point. There would be mistakes ahead, and days when I wished I could crawl back into bed, but I was on my way to becoming a surgeon, and that was grand.

Surgeons of my generation taught ourselves how to do a lot of things. The expectations of surgery residents and their supervisors have changed since then. My residents rarely, if ever, do their first procedure unsupervised, and most of them wouldn't want to be left to themselves even if I was prepared to leave them. However, apropos of Dr. Julie Meadow's comments in Chapter 5, there is an extraordinary sense of accomplishment that comes from pushing beyond your safety zone and realizing that your judgment and skill are the sole determiners of a successful outcome.

When I moved from the University of Sydney to UC Davis, I found myself amongst an awe-inspiring array of discipline specialists. And although I thought I had a pretty good handle on surgery, I discovered that different veterinary schools had very different approaches to some of the simplest things. The older you get, though, the harder it is to acknowledge that someone else's approach might be better – or at least as good.

I learned a technique (we referred to it as the Penn technique in honor of the PennWees) for placing three sutures in the mesenteric aspect of an intestinal anastomosis and thus avoiding dehiscence at that vulnerable site. I learned that rectal pull-through could be equally effective as a dorsal approach in the majority of cases. I learned that you can take excellent liver biopsies using a skin punch. In some of these cases, it hadn't even occurred to me that there might be a better way of doing things. I certainly would not have thought to ask for advice about them, when I had taught myself to do such a good job already.

More recently fledged surgeons often have similarly concrete ideas on how something should be done, but will explain them as, "This is how I was trained." I hope, as they grow up with stricter surgical supervision, our trainees retain the ability to be creative and push their own boundaries.

My first TECA took almost three hours. If Missy came to me tomorrow, I expect I could complete the surgery in about 30 minutes. I would like to think I am no less meticulous, or no less careful, and my results seem to support that. But what am I doing differently now, to what I was doing before? How did I become a faster surgeon? We know that time in surgery makes a difference; both to anesthetic and surgical complication rates. But how can we reduce surgical time without compromising our standards?

Professor Chris Bellenger, my primary surgery supervisor, is an elegant man; meticulous in his demeanor, approach, and behavior. He taught me many things, perhaps the most memorable being that surgery has its own unique choreography. When lecturing on how to become a surgeon, I point out that every surgery is a series of steps: making an incision, separating soft tissues, ligating, anastomosing, reinforcing, then suturing. Imagine a novice skier learning to do basic turns. Then imagine the skier beginning to link those turns, faster and faster, until they progress down the slope at high speed, but in complete control, in a seemingly effortless transition from one turn to the next. Chris Bellenger emphasized economy of motion in surgery; if you reach for an instrument, make sure you know where it is. Make sure it is the correct instrument, and think about what you actually plan to do with it. Which band of tissue will you cut, and which will you tease apart? If you ensure that every action during surgery moves you closer to the end goal, you can save enormous amounts of time.

Following multiple successful ear canal ablations as a resident, I found myself as a new surgery Faculty. Sadly, because of funding cuts and internal politics, a number of long-standing Faculty departed, and for a while I was the only soft tissue surgeon. My self-instruction would have to continue.

Barkley McMullen was a six-year-old Rottweiler with chronic otitis externa and bilateral otitis media. Like Missy, the Afghan, his ear canals were still patent and his disease seemed focused in the tympanic bullae. I decided to treat him with bilateral ventral bulla osteotomies (VBO), rather than ear canal ablations. I had done one VBO on a cat a year previously with a visiting surgeon. He told me that – in his view – this was a procedure where it was better not to know the anatomy. A quick look at the textbook revealed a frightening array of named structures running on either side of the bulla, and you did not want to be thinking about them while you were cutting.

"Palpate the bulla through the skin," he said, demonstrating on the skinny cat's neck. "And dissect straight onto it. Make sure your plane of dissection is in a craniocaudal direction, and you should push the important structures apart, rather than transecting them."

I couldn't help myself, I had to know what the "important" structures were. Miller's told me that they were the internal carotid artery, glossopharyngeal and hypoglossal nerves. The visiting surgeon was correct, structures like those are hard to put out of your mind when you are approaching them with sharp instruments.

We anesthetized the Rottweiler, and I went off to scrub while the surgery techs laid him on his back and prepped his neck. I had purchased some colorful socks sporting tropical fish, and decided to make them my "lucky" surgery socks. Barkley would be their first test. My surgery resident draped in the site and had the instruments on the surgery table neatly laid out and ready for me. Seamless.

"We'll start by palpating the bullae," I said, interrogating the site with one finger. Gentle probing turned to more vigorous poking, as Barkley's thick Rottweiler throat failed to yield its secrets. I palpated something hard, but couldn't be sure whether it was larynx or hyoid bone. As I poked, his neck flexed, his chin elevated, and his retropharyngeal structures migrated away from me.

"Did we extend his head over a sandbag?" I asked.

The tech and resident looked blank.

I poked around in the hope of locating something (anything) that I could identify, and finally found the angle of the mandible. I realized that the drapes had been placed caudal to the larynx. Fortunately, Barkley had been clipped and prepped right up between the bodies of the mandible and I was able to reposition the drapes cranially. I calculated the level of his larynx and pushed harder with my finger. Barkley's head twisted to one side.

"Did we tie his head down with tape?" I asked. Again, no response.

Realizing that palpating a Rottweiler's bulla was a different prospect from that of a cat, I had the resident hold Barkley's head steady as I made a skin incision lateral to the larynx and medial to where I thought his linguofacial vein might run.

"We'll dissect in a little deeper," I said, "and then try palpating again." This simple strategy failed also. I found myself dissecting deeper and deeper into the dog's neck with little real idea of where I was headed. I fell back on the hope that if I dissected longitudinally, I might part, rather than tear, those vital structures I had read about. As the surgical incision became deeper, it turned into more of a tunnel, and the diagram from Miller's flashed like a neon sign in my head. I was too scared to incise anything I could not see, and hence my access was getting tighter and tighter. I called for Gelpi retractors, but they were too narrow and sharp. Weitlaner's were too bulky. I positioned them, but then I couldn't fit my finger in to palpate. I took them out again. Tried Langenbeck hand-held retractors. Began humming. This was not turning out the way I had anticipated.

Eventually, I palpated a hard, dome-shaped structure at the base of Barkley's skull. Finally!

"There we go," I told the resident happily.

"Can I have a feel?"

"Of course."

The resident poked at the general area.

"Do you feel it?"

He poked some more. Moved his finger around. His expression suggested that he really, really wanted to be able to say yes, but …

"No."

"Let me try again," I said. I inserted my finger but could not find that welcome protruberance. "It was right here …" I felt something spongy and cord-like. It had a pulse. I palpated some more and found the raised bony structure again. "I'll dissect onto it and you can have another feel," I said.

I began digging in the deep hole. I found myself in a muscle belly, but could feel bone right underneath it. What I was expecting was to break through the periosteum and watch the soft tissues gradually peel back, revealing the shiny white dome of the tympanic bulla. Instead, I got some venous bleeding, and more muscle. I dissected further.

Craniocaudal, I told myself. *Don't think about the internal carotid artery.*

It was getting hot in the OR. I started to sweat. I began wondering how bad the signs of hypoglossal paralysis were likely to be. Not something I had discussed with the owner, being so focused on damage to the vestibular apparatus or failure to resolve the infection. I replaced the Langenbeck retractors with malleable ribbon retractors. Too thick. I adjusted the surgery lights and repalpated the mandibles. The tough fibrous tissue would not yield to my right-angled forceps. I really, *really* didn't want to cut anything, so I picked and worried at the tissues until they shredded. Finally, I exposed a shelf of bone. The resident loaded a Steinmann pin into a hand chuck.

I felt the need to inject a little light humor. As I twisted the sharp point into the bone, I said, "If you're going to drill holes in the base of the skull, you really want to know you are drilling through the right thing."

Nervous laughter from the students. I felt sick. The point of the pin engaged, I pushed harder, and popped straight through. This was a surprise; based on the radiographs I expected the bone to be half an inch thick.

"We're in," I said to the students, who couldn't see anything of the surgery site.

The resident handed me a curette. I inserted it gently, expecting a rush of pus. All I got was blood.

"Suction!"

The bleeding settled and I probed deeper with the curette. I was expecting to hit the dorsal wall of the bulla, but it sunk into something soft. I didn't let on to my assistants, but I honestly thought I had found the brainstem. When the curette emerged, it trailed shreds of something suspiciously like muscle.

"That's odd," I mumbled.

I came to the nauseating realization that I was completely lost inside this dog's head. I asked the surgery techs to find a skeleton so I could work out which particular bony prominence I might have bored through. I still don't know for sure what it was, but at the time I convinced

myself it was the occipital condyle. My "lucky" surgery socks were failing their first test.

By now, we had been in surgery for an hour and a half and I was no closer to my goal. We'll talk in Chapter 10 about the various ways I have learned to find my way back on track when I am lost in surgery, but for now I will tell you that I did eventually find Barkley's tympanic bulla. It was about a centimeter thick and I ended up attacking it with a burr. The surgery took almost four hours, yielded a scant amount of hyperplastic mucosa, and necessitated having two additional students scrub in as they successively dropped like flies. Barkley recovered without complication, responded temporarily but then relapsed, and had his ear canals removed about six months later. I never wore those socks again.

Experiences with patients like Barkley make me contemplate what I have learned about how to be a faster and more effective surgeon, without compromising safety.

As Professor Bellenger demonstrated, fast surgery is efficient surgery. We lost time in Barkley's surgery by not placing him correctly on the table. I should have spent a few minutes discussing the preparation and draping with my team, maybe even helping to position him so I knew I would be properly orientated when I scrubbed in. Getting the drapes in the right place. Working out which landmarks I needed for navigation.

I learned early on to value my time at the scrub sink as an aid to personal preparation. For some reason, people are much less likely to bother you with other issues while you are scrubbing for surgery. They will bowl in during a delicate adrenal dissection to ask whether Rufus needs to be fed at 6 p.m. or 8 p.m., or interrupt a liver resection to let you know that Mrs. Farrell broke her toe and won't be coming in tomorrow morning, but the scrub sink seems to be a protected zone. It is one reason that I never moved completely to using alcohol-based hand wipes, even thought the evidence suggests that – used properly – they are just as good as the old-fashioned 10-minute scrub. That 10-minute scrub gives me an opportunity to brush off concerns from the other side of the sterile red line, compose myself, focus on what is about to come, and think through the procedure step by step, making sure we have made the right preparations, selected the right instruments, written all the biopsy samples we want to take on a "shopping list," made sure we have the right-sized catheters, suture material, and other disposables. Athletes talk about being "in the zone" when they compete; forcing themselves to focus on the here and now, and block extraneous stimuli. The 10-minute scrub is a great – possibly your only – chance to get into the zone.

Remember that I likened surgery to skiing earlier in this chapter, so let's explore the athletic analogy a little further. While taking a private ski lesson just a few years ago, I asked my instructor the best way to prepare myself for skiing when I spent so little time in the snowfields.

"Well, apart from making sure you are physically fit, you can imagine the moves in your head," he replied.

This seemed ludicrous; how could you imagine something as physical as skiing?

"I now it sounds crazy," he said, "but try it tonight."

I did, when I was lying in bed waiting for sleep. I pictured myself negotiating a steep slope; how did I position my shoulders, where was I looking, how was I shifting my weight? In no time at all, my feet were twitching with each imaginary turn as I sailed down a virtual black run.

I decided to try it with surgery. As time went on, I became able to visualize a surgery in my head. How would the tissues look as I incised them; how well would they separate; what visualization would my approach afford; how securely could I suture them; and how well would they heal? Try it yourself. If it works, this is something else you can do during your surgical preparation time; not only will it get you into a suitable frame of mind, but it might remind you of something you could otherwise have overlooked.

With Barkley's surgery, I definitely could have prepared better for the actual procedure.

Practiced the surgery on a cadaver, looked at a skeleton ahead of time, even brought it into the OR proactively if I thought I might need it. Thought about the best way to ensure I was on the right track while dissecting.

I ended up with a surgery table cluttered with instruments I did not use. This wasted time as the techs scrambled to find something I tried and then discarded and, at the end of the day, someone had to wash, repackage, and resterilize.

After an hour or more of fruitless activity, we become flustered and frustrated. Our assistants become tired and lose focus or, if they haven't slept well the night before, or eaten lunch, may manifest the strain by passing out. As time goes on, our chance of doing more harm than good gets higher and higher. We are likely to make hasty decisions, rash moves, lean down and pick a hemostat from the trash without thinking.

Twenty-five years later, when I find myself in a similar situation – which I do, as you will see in a later chapter – I try to regroup. I take some time out. Clean up the instrument table (Figure 9.1). Wash my surgery gloves with cool saline. Take some deep breaths, do some stretches. I talk through the dilemma with my surgical team and knock around ideas, and try to refocus. I talk to my anesthetist; they are a part of the team, too, and will be wondering what is going on: is everything okay, should they be worried?

We review our plan and talk about what could we do differently in the next phase of the surgery that might help us to be more successful. Although it seems counterintuitive to stop and chat when you are taking too long in surgery, a strategic break when people are getting tired and stressed can save time in the long run. And bringing your team into it means that you do not go it alone, and they are not subjected to the painful process of watching you do it.

In years of training surgeons, I have seen both ends of the spectrum; approaches that simultaneously epitomize and contravene Halstead's principles. I have seen surgeons who were

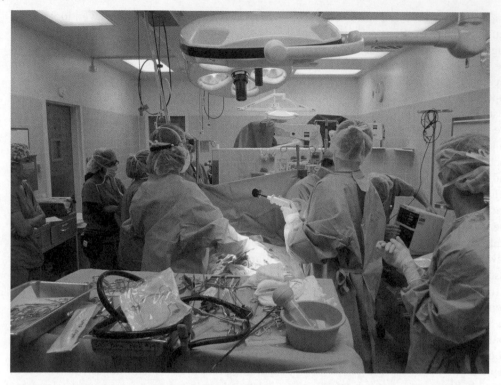

Figure 9.1 Demonstrating what *not* to do with your surgical table. Having to sift through muddled and dirty instruments wastes valuable time.

meticulous to a fault; ligating every small bleeder, agonizing over every strand of tissue before cutting it, poking, pulling, and rethinking, and worrying. And the surgeons who seem to cut first and ask questions later; boring into a back or a leg with seemingly little concern. Surgeons who ask advice from everyone and anyone, and those who don't ask anyone.

The ideal surgeon manages a balance between the two.

10

"It Didn't Look Like That on Paper!"

When Textbooks Let Us Down

Between finishing my PhD and starting my surgery residency, I spent a year working in Sydney's south-west. It was a one-and-a-half doctor, small animal practice, owned by a mid-career vet I had met at Continuing Education events. He always asked good questions of the lecturers and, despite the relatively humble nature of his practice, seemed committed to providing high-quality care. The practice was in an industrial area, nestled between two major roads. Socioeconomically, the surrounding suburbs were middle class at best, and the clientele very careful with their money. Our patient population included a large subset of dusty, junkyard dogs bearing stud collars and called Killer. Despite their intimidating appearance, some of these dogs were quite friendly. But many were not.

Ruthie was an intact middle-aged Boxer cross with allergic dermatitis and teats around her ankles, who had undoubtedly begat multiple generations of "Killers." She arrived with a history of drooling and lethargy. The owner claimed no knowledge of her toileting history ("What's *feces*?") or whether she was vomiting ("She lives in my truck yard"). After examining Ruthie, my fingers were coated in a greasy black film. I was suspicious of something in her abdomen but could not be sure, and recommended blood work.

I was off-duty when the results came back. Ruthie's clinical signs continued and another vet working part-time in the practice palpated her abdomen again and diagnosed an intestinal foreign body. When the vet rang to get permission for surgery, Ruthie's owner requested euthanasia.

My boss spoke to me the next day. "We didn't learn anything from the blood tests that we couldn't see on physical exam. But we could have put that money towards surgery."

I didn't know how to respond. It made sense. But how was I to know that Ruthie had a treatable surgical disease rather than garbage guts, or some weird intoxication? It seemed reasonable to investigate further in order to confirm the best course of action. In a veterinary teaching hospital, we would do blood tests, abdominal sonography, and probably also a chest X-ray before making any real commitments regarding diagnosis and prognosis. Here was a catch-22: how could we be comfortable taking the next step without baseline data?

I would love to say this dilemma no longer exists in the modern age of veterinary practice. But it does and vets across the world deal with it every day. The owner will approve an ultrasound, but not a CT; they agree to blood work, but not a radiograph. Mr. Blakeney won't pay for any tests beyond a consultation. Wherever the buck stops, though, we have to try to do the basics well: history, physical examination, evaluation of the patient in light of the available evidence. And at some point in the process we then have to trust ourselves to do the best we can with the information we have.

The textbook may tell us the next step, and it is tempting to keep ordering tests until the diagnosis is completely beyond doubt, but at some point we will find ourselves on our own, and then we have to rely on our own innate judgment.

Pitfalls in Veterinary Surgery, First Edition. Edited by Geraldine B. Hunt.
© 2017 John Wiley & Sons, Inc. Published 2017 by John Wiley & Sons, Inc.

For patients such as Ruthie, who do not come in with a diagnosis (for whom you cannot search the index and flip to the appropriate page), the textbooks may have to wait until you have found enough clues to tell you which chapter to read.

Were I to see Ruthie again, I would still do blood work. But perhaps I would limit it to things I could check easily in the consulting room: packed cell volume (PCV), total protein, glucose, blood urea nitrogen. Then if I was really concerned about abdominal disease and an ultrasound was out of the question, I would take an abdominal X-ray. After that, it would be up to me and the owner to decide whether we were comfortable going further on the strength of the available information.

Textbooks can be our best friends and our greatest challenges. Riffling through *Small Animal Surgery* to discover a neat description of our patient's seemingly exotic problem can be a great comfort. Confronting its multiple chapters and kilograms of detailed knowledge when we begin studying for Boards is intimidating, to say the least.

As we move deeper into the digital age, physical textbooks feature less in our day-to-day lives. Early in my career, I had one or perhaps two key reference books for each of the major disciplines, and everything in them was gospel. Textbooks were my constant companions; each new edition promising a myriad of fresh and exciting information.

Now we have many competing "oracles" in each discipline. New titles and editions come out regularly, and for the most up-to-date thoughts and ideas we turn to the internet.

For blow-by-blow details of surgical anatomy, however, we still resort to the old faithfuls with whom we grew up. The catch is, we are using a two-dimensional medium to gather three-dimensional information. Add to this the fact that medical illustrators must draw cartoon-like images to emphasize salient features, and we find that the picture in the textbook can look very different from the bloody, oily, tattered, and generally obscure surgical field we encounter in real life.

Coming straight from advanced training in thoracic surgery to small animal practice, with limited diagnostics, and clients who expected as much treatment as possible for their money – ironic in light of my later failure with Ruthie – my surgical skills were greeted with great excitement. The Friday before my first day alone in the practice, my boss phoned.

"I've got a great surgical case for you on Monday!"

"What is it?"

"A Dachshund with a bilateral perineal hernia."

As I mentioned in Chapter 9, my expertise in the chest did not necessarily translate to other regions, and the perineum could not be much further from my comfort zone. Nevertheless, I replied, "Great; can't wait!"

I studied Slatter's *Textbook of Small Animal Surgery* over the weekend. Memorized the musculature of the perineal diaphragm. Ran through the various steps of the surgery in my mind, and chose the sutures that I would use.

How hard could this be?

Rommel was waiting for me on Monday morning, having been dropped off bright and early by his elderly owner.

"Let's have a look," I said to Raquel, the nurse. Raquel tucked Rommel's head under one arm (his mouth was uncomfortably close to her ample bosom, but presumably she already knew and trusted this dog because I have to assume you only make that mistake once). She swung Rommel around for me to examine his nether regions.

It was a horrible sight. A greatly swollen dome beneath, and partly engulfing, his tail base. The reddened and stretched anus looked remarkably like a mouth in the process of screaming. Rather than emitting a wail, however, this mouth drooled an eccentric rivulet of liquid feces. I attempted to insert my gloved finger into Rommel's rectum, but could only enter a lateral sacculation just beneath the skin, at which point he growled and flicked his head, and Raquel let him go.

"Right," I said. "Let's get him anesthetized."

And work things out from there, I thought, but did not say, as this was not going entirely to plan.

Raquel wrestled Rommel (who now wore a muzzle) as I found a vein and anesthetized him. We clipped the back end, evacuated the liquid feces (he had been on liberal quantities of stool softener), and placed a purse string suture in the anus. After castrating him, I positioned him in sternal recumbency over the rolled-up towel that was our version of a perineal stand. Mentally reviewing the pertinent page of the surgical text as I applied scalpel blade to skin, I made my first para-anal incision. I went part way through the dermis; deep enough to cause bleeding, but not deep enough for the incision to separate sufficiently for me to see anything in order to clamp it.

Deep breath.

I extended the incision. And got a rush of turbid, foul-smelling liquid. For a moment, I thought I had perforated his rectum, but quickly realized it was his anal sac.

Doh!

I had forgotten about anal sacs during the preparation. I mention this because I *still* forget anal sacs to this day, and if I don't remember to flush and evacuate them, I can't really expect my techs or students to do so. *Always check the anal sacs when you are doing surgery around the perineum.*

This could have been a major hurdle, but fortunately I have a surgical temperament. After a moment's shock, and feeling both guilty for the surgical contamination I had just created, and foolish because I had not predicted this outcome, I excised the offending anal sac and proceeded with the rest of the surgery.

I had an optimistic idea that once I cut into the hernial sac, the muscles of the perineal diaphragm would present themselves and it would be a simple matter to place the sutures and tie them. Things unfolded a little differently.

Once through the skin, I encountered multiple vessels and string-like structures approaching the anus. I realized that I knew very little about the pudendal and perineal nerves and arteries. Were these them? I dissected dorsal and ventral to these structures and encountered a bulging gray membrane. The hernia sac! I

tentatively punctured it and jumped back as yellow fluid jetted out. I could only think of one source of yellow fluid, and realized I was not entirely sure where this dog's bladder was. I had assumed it was in the abdomen, but had I just perforated it?

Fortunately, the yellow flood was followed by a tongue of diaphanous membrane that I recognized as omentum. *Phew!*

Nothing I had read in the textbook really prepared me for the messy reality of this surgery. The omentum contained small nodules and cysts. I burst the cysts and pushed the nodules back into the abdomen. Consisting of organizing hematomas and areas of saponification, these objects are common in long-standing perineal hernias (Figure 10.1).

Having incised through the skin, and opened the hernia sac, I now faced a surgical site that was bleeding at several points, oozing abdominal fluid, with the anatomic structures completely obscured by fat, escaping omentum, and fibrous adhesions. Somewhere in this mess was the pudendal nerve, artery, and vein, which made me reluctant to do much in the way of dissection. But if I didn't dissect, how could I identify the muscles that I needed to put my sutures through?

In addition to the two lateral hernias, Rommel had a large ventral component. His entire anus was separated from its perineal support and had migrated caudal to his tuber ischia, making it difficult to use them as a landmark for incision and dissection. In order to repair these hernias, I would have to implement some form of ventral support in addition to the lateral sutures. The natural thing seemed to be to suture the left and right obturator muscles together beneath the anus. In order to increase my exposure, and in the hope that the structures of the left side would be easier to identify, I packed some gauze into the large hole on the right side, and repeated the surgical approach on the left side. Having decompressed the hernia from the right side, I did not encounter the same gush of fluid or inexorable slither of balled-up omentum. Instead, I found myself in a cavity much more

(A) (B)

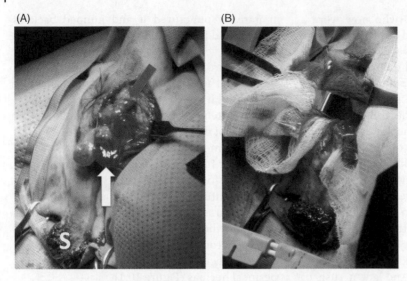

Figure 10.1 (A) Mess of cystic and saponified omentum (white arrow) emerging from perineal hernia incision. A small organizing hematoma is also present, for good measure (gray arrow). Note that the scrotum (S) has been included in the surgical field to allow a castration via a caudal approach. (B) Using surgical gauze and Langenbeck retractors to provide hemostasis and hold tissues apart to assist visualization while placing sutures.

like I had been expecting. I still could not see the muscles I was supposed to suture, but at least I wasn't shouldering my way through viscera. Wary following my experience with the right anal sac, I had made my incision quite lateral to the anus, but with some medial dissection I was able to expose the external anal sphincter. I was reluctant to dissect the soft tissues from the ischium, but palpated the bilateral tuber ischia and followed them medially to the concave ischiatic arch. It seemed there was solid tissue in there to incorporate in my repair. I decided to start the repair on this side, and move back to the other side when I had a better idea of the general anatomy.

This was the first time I observed that, with bilateral disease, one side is usually "better" or "easier" than the other side. This is definitely true of perineal hernias and, strangely, often of total ear canal ablations. If you get lucky (or clever) you can attack the easy side first, and thus gain confidence for the more difficult one. In Rommell's case I did it the other way round, but in accidentally stumbling upon the phenomenon, he helped me develop a strategy for the future.

I had placed a suture through the ventral anal sphincter (being careful to avoid the palpably distended anal sac) and was about to grasp a deep bite of the tissue occupying the ischiatic arch when something stopped me. Being unfamiliar with the anatomy of the area, my mind had been processing the potential hazards, and suddenly reminded me of something important.

The urethra runs over the caudal ischium, separating from the penis and traversing the floor of the pelvic cavity. Had I placed my sutures deep into the ischiatic arch, I could have perforated or even occluded the pelvic urethra. Relieved at this lucky escape, I began palpating the notch in order to identify, and thus avoid, the urethra. Unfortunately, the urethra is soft, and although it is possible to palpate it more cranially, surrounded by its fleshy urethralis muscle, it is quite hard to feel as it curves around the ischium. I made a mental note to place a urinary catheter for my next bilateral perineal hernia, so I would always know exactly where the urethra ran.

The other issue was that Rommell's prostate was large and cystic, and hard to differentiate from the cystic and nodular omentum in the hernia sac. I poked everything cranially, but also thought it would be a good idea in future to establish the position and structure of the prostate before surgery. I read later that the peritoneal reflection is closely associated with the prostate, and it contains the important neurovascular structures to the neck of the bladder. Damaging the peritoneal reflection can lead to urinary incontinence, and is probably the reason some dogs leak urine after bilateral perineal hernia repair. Being aware of these anatomic features, and being judicious with dissection in the general region, should reduce the risk of this complication.

I did eventually complete Rommell's surgery, but I never confidently identified the coccygeus muscle, and my sutures did not result in a solid repair of the pelvic diaphragm. The owner was delighted with the result, but to this day I don't know whether I really made a difference to Rommel, or whether the owner's satisfaction was purely placebo. I did learn, however, that if I were ever to perform this surgery competently, I would have to learn a lot more about the local anatomy, and become far more confident with soft tissue dissection.

The last thing I learned from Rommell's case – which stood me in great stead when tackling one of the cases in Chapter 17 – was that although a hernia repair using the available musculature can be extremely robust, the muscles tear easily if you place an undue amount of force on individual sutures. I realized that I had to encourage the muscles to come together and ensure there was minimal tension as they healed, rather than forcing them into apposition. I don't respond well to being forced, and neither do living tissues; somehow, we find a way of making our displeasure known. In my case, it takes the form of instant hostility or sullen disobedience. A delicate muscle shreds or necroses. The end result is the same.

Once I realized this, the size and type of suture material became less important, as long as I chose something that would maintain its holding power well into the wound maturation phase (i.e., at least six weeks). Using a thick suture that

was far stronger than the native tissues was just as likely to result in tissue trauma as it was tightened. Most tissues heal well, if only we treat them politely.

Despite what I just said about the deficiencies of "cartoons," the diagrams in textbooks highlight important features of a surgical procedure in a way that can be far more relevant than words. In some respects, they are like waypoints in the journey of each particular operation, rather like the street view in Google Earth™. They are saying "this is what it should look like when you reach this particular point." But they don't necessarily help you with the nitty gritty logistics of actually getting to that point. How do you negotiate the four-way stop sign? Is it safe to drive through the water that has flooded the dip beneath the railway bridge? What is the speed limit along this stretch of road?

Incising through the hernia sac and entering Rummell's pelvic cavity was simply the first step towards the waypoint depicted in the surgical text, in which the anal sphincter, internal obturator, and coccygeus muscles were neatly exposed in preparation for insertion of sutures. Somehow, I had to separate, excise, or otherwise move the fat and fibrous tissue without damaging the vital structures I knew to be nestled among it. How would I decide what could be safely ligated and cut, and when it would be better to push things aside than dissect through them? I didn't work this out in time for Rommell, but it did come to me in subsequent cases as I became more familiar with the surgical anatomy.

I started by reviewing what I knew of anatomy in general. First, the neural structures coming out to the skin are largely sensory, and there is a rich collateral sensory innervation in most parts of the body, so dividing structures from a region of skin and superficial subcutis is unlikely to lead to major complications. The ischiatic tuberosities form critical landmarks in perineal hernia surgery. In a patient with a normal perineal diaphragm, the anus is in a plane slightly cranial to the palpable tuberosities. Caudal migration of the anus suggests separation or at least weakness of the perineal diaphragm, even when a hernia is not obviously palpable. This is especially common in cats, which often display fecal retention just cranial to the anus as a result of perineal laxity, without the classic defect of perineal hernia (see Chapter 17).

I palpated Rommell's ischiatic tuberosity and concluded that it would be safe to dissect the subcutaneous tissue and fat in a plane between the skin and the bony prominence. I thus exposed the caudal edge of the ischium, which allowed me to incise the periosteum and start to lift it (and the internal obturator) from the floor of the pelvic canal. Gentle elevation of the muscle, and focused sharp dissection of the dense fibrous tissue lateral and medial to the muscle directly off the bone allowed me to mobilize the internal obturators without doing any dissection in the fatty tissue dorsal and cranial to the ischium. Exposing the anal sphincter was fairly straightforward once I convinced myself that ligating and diving the superficial blood vessels was unlikely to cause major morbidity. Now came the issue of the coccygeus muscles. Dogs get perineal hernias because of muscle atrophy and weakness; therefore it is unrealistic to expect their coccygeus muscle to leap out of the surgical field and ask to be sutured. But when I looked into the surgical site, all I could see was a large fat pad. I knew the coccygeus must be in there somewhere, but I could not feel it, and I had a strong gut feeling that if I started to dissect I would hit the pudendal nerve, or even worse, the sciatic!

I mulled over what I knew of the coccygeus muscle which was, sadly, very little. Its name provided a clue. "Coccygeus" suggested it had some relationship to the vertebrae of the tail. Perhaps if I moved the tail, the muscle might stretch and be easier to palpate. I did exactly that, and the combination of palpating from inside the pelvic cavity–hernia ring, and elevating the tail, allowed me to feel the soft tubular muscle directly caudomedial to the sacrotuberous ligament. In most species, muscle has a distinctly different feel to fat, so palpation can be very helpful in surgery. It also helps when choosing the leanest lamb roast in the supermarket.

I could feel Rommel's coccygeus muscle, but it was still obscured by fat. I thought further about the anatomy. I knew the sciatic ran cranial to the sacrotuberous ligament, so if I restricted my dissection to the caudal edge I was probably safe. I was still not entirely sure about the pudendal, but I knew it came through the pelvic canal, so if I stayed relatively lateral I should be able to avoid that, too. I settled on a plane of dissection designed to separate the intrapelvic fat pad from the subcutaneous fat caudal and lateral to the sacrotuberous ligament, directly over the region in which the coccygeus was palpably stretching when I extended the tail. Miraculously, the tissues separated with minimal dissection and I was rewarded by a layer of glistening gray fascia overlying the tell-tale ligamentous striations of the coccygeus muscle. Having identified the muscle belly, it was a far less nerve-wracking process to elevate the fat from it dorsally and ventrally and expose a long enough segment for suturing.

Even this description, though – breaking the process of dissection into bite-sized pieces – has glossed over the challenge of holding back the slithering omentum, and preventing the subcutaneous fat and skin from rolling medially to block your view. Strategic placement of retractors is critical; this is not a surgery you can easily do on your own. After years of trial and error, I settled on a combination of techniques. A dynamic self-retaining device that allows for circumferential retraction (e.g., the LoneStar retractor[1]) is enormously helpful (Figure 10.2). I use moistened surgical sponges to push the viscera back into the pelvic cavity, and hold them in place with a malleable ribbon or Langenbeck retractor (Figure 10.1B). Ideally, the sponges should be secured by a mosquito forcep or a surgical suture, to ensure they do not disappear into the peritoneal cavity, and you should *always do a sponge count* before closing the hernia ring. Once the sponge has been placed, you can move your retractors medially or laterally to expose

---

1 Cooper Surgical, CT, USA.

the relevant musculature. In recent years, I have even taken to placing the patients in dorsal recumbency, which facilitates conjoint procedures such as colopexy and castration, improves visualization of the coccygeus muscle, and relieves your assistant of having to keep the tail up and out of the way when the tail-tie comes off (Figure 10.3).

The unfortunate thing about learning anatomy from textbooks, or even from computer programs, is that they are forced to provide a two-dimensional representation of a three-dimensional surgical field. I've spent countless hours in the anatomy lab, working with students who clutch a formalin-stained print-out of an anatomic illustration but fail to find any of the structures so neatly outlined in black and white. One of the biggest traps is to determine whether you have a medial or lateral view. Do you really expect the femoral artery to be running *lateral* to the femur? Does that make sense in any biologic system? The other way textbooks confuse us is by conveniently removing or erasing important overlying structures. Yes, it looks as if the sciatic nerve is the next thing you encounter after incising the subcutaneous tissue, but only if you have also resected the biceps femoris muscle. Gaining an appreciation of the three-dimensional nature of a surgical field, and the geometric relationship of one structure to another is critical. You may be lost in a surgical field, but if you know the sciatic nerve runs cranial to the sacrotuberous ligament, and you can palpate the sacrotuberous ligament, then you can focus your dissection in a safe area. If you can palpate the tuber ischium, you know that elevating the obturator muscle by peeling the periosteum from the bone will allow you to reflect the vital structures away from harm.

I call this strategy *working from the known to the unknown*.

Recall the last chapter when I lost my way deep in Barkley's retropharynx while searching

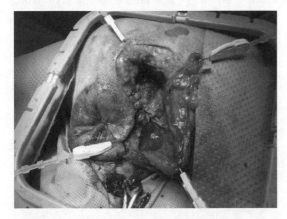

Figure 10.2 Elasticized self-retaining retractor being used for perineal hernia repair in another patient.

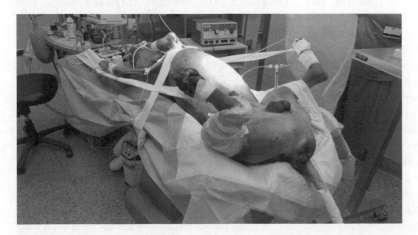

Figure 10.3 Dog positioned in dorsal recumbency for perineal hernia repair.

for his tympanic bulla. I had read the descriptions, studied the illustrations, and conjured a neat mental image of what to expect, but when none of these things matched up in reality, I was completely stuck. I had already bored through an inappropriate bony shelf near the base of his skull, and had a narrow escape when I found myself burrowing through another muscle. But I was not going to be so lucky next time, so I was getting desperate. I knew of one palpable landmark – the angular process of the mandible – but it was so distant from the bulla itself as to be almost useless apart from positioning of the primary incision. The bulla is smooth and dome-shaped, which is helpful when you palpate it, but doesn't stand out easily from the surrounding structures in a patient with a thick neck. I needed something that was both easily palpable and also in close proximity to the bulla itself. The wing of the atlas provided another mechanism for orienting me in the general region, but it still would not lead me exactly where I needed to go.

"Can you bring in Miller's?" I asked the tech, referring to the *Anatomy of the Dog.*

Searching isolated anatomic structures for inspiration was not especially helpful, but reviewing the regional anatomy was; in particular, the diagram depicting the hyoid apparatus. I could palpate the hyoid bones lateral to the pharynx, arising from the basihyoid and extending dorsally on either side of the pharynx. The illustration reminded me (if I had ever known this) that the stylohyoid bone passed ventral to the ear canal and lateral to the tympanic bulla before articulating with the skull by means of the tympanohyoid cartilage. If I followed the hyoid bones dorsally, they would eventually lead me right to the bulla. I did that, and confirmation of the anatomic position gave me confidence to dissect through the thin musculature surrounding the bulla. I exposed a smooth dome that looked and felt just like I thought the bulla should. However, following my experience with drilling through the other bony shelf, I needed more proof.

What else leads to the bulla? I wondered.

My second lightbulb moment might have presented itself earlier had I not been so terrified. There was another structure as obvious and wide as the Pacific Highway that would take me straight into the bulla: the external ear canal! Which would have been fine, had I draped it into the surgical field.

I sent the surgery tech under the drapes to locate and flush the ear canal, and then repositioned the drapes on either side to give me access to the ears. The resultant surgical contamination seemed a small price to pay. I inserted a Kelly clamp into the ear canal and manipulated it to the level of the eardrum. Placing my finger just lateral to the stylohyoid bone, I could feel the tips of the Kellys as I wiggled them up and down, confirming that the dome-shaped bone was indeed the bulla.

Finally!

I became very grateful for this reassurance as the bulla proved at least a centimeter thick and I needed the air drill to penetrate it. Imagine the last time you were caught in grid-locked traffic; running late, without a roadmap; and you will have an inkling of how it feels to bore through the skull while uncertain of what you will find on the other side.

Scamp was a middle-aged Cocker Spaniel who presented to his local veterinarian with dysphagia. The vet palpated a mass caudal to the left mandible. The tentative diagnosis was a retropharyngeal abscess secondary to foreign body migration. Fine needle aspiration failed to yield pus, but it seemed logical to explore the area to confirm the diagnosis and treat Scamp's problem. An incision was made over the most obvious part of the swelling, caudal to the mandible and lateral to the pharynx. After a substantial amount of dissection, which necessitated ligation of a series of large blood vessels, the vet was able to remove several masses. Histopathology confirmed them to be a normal submandibular lymph node, the mandibular salivary gland, and another, neoplastic, node; presumably the retropharyngeal.

Scamp presented to me for an opinion about whether further surgery to obtain clean surgical margins was feasible. He had a facial droop with a dirty rope of saliva hanging from his mouth, his tongue protruded, and he had severe Horner's syndrome on the operated side. Biopsying his retropharyngeal lymph node had come at a high cost.

I broke the news to the owner that I doubted I would be able to obtain a surgical margin without causing significant additional morbidity.

"Oh, we already knew that."

If that were the case, I wondered why they had come to me?

"Our vet was keen for us to see you," they offered. "He was very happy he could get the lymph node out at all. He did a great job!"

Looking at Scamp, I wasn't entirely sure I agreed. I had never removed a retropharyngeal lymph node, and wondered how I would approach it when the time came. Happy as Scamp's owners were with his outcome, surely there was a better way?

When the time came for me to work out an approach to the region, I wasn't chasing a retropharyngeal lymph node (although there have been plenty since).

Vegemite was a young adult Staffy who had been involved in an altercation with his neighbour, Bob, a large Rottweiler. Bob had grabbed Vegemite around the throat and delivered a good shaking. The deep punctures on either side of Vegemite's neck bled substantially, but Vegemite responded well to placement of a pressure bandage, analgesia, and prophylactic antibiotics. Over the next 48 hours, though, his face began to swell and he developed a fever. Vegemite was referred to us on suspicion of having a cervical abscess, possibly from esophageal trauma (Figure 10.4A).

When I examined Vegemite's neck, it was a mess. The whole left side was swollen and edematous. The skin was bruised and indurated, and it was almost impossible to palpate the normal landmarks. How was I going to explore it without damaging any number of vital structures? I flashed back on Scamp's drooping mouth and prolapsed third eyelid, and predicted similar complications for Vegemite.

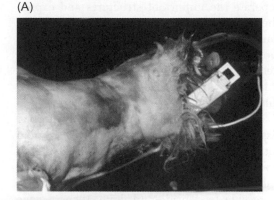

(A)

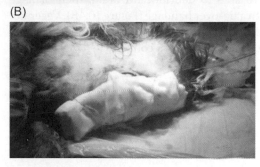

(B)

Figure 10.4 (A) Dog with extensive neck trauma caused by bite wounds (dorsal recumbency). (B) The same dog in left lateral recumbency, demonstrating a tie-over bandage for open drainage following exploration and debridement through a ventral midline incision.

It was tempting to incise through the region of greatest trauma, in the expectation that the major pathology would be focused there, but I hesitated.

"What is the safest way into Vegemite's neck?" I asked the students.

Understandably, they had little to offer.

"Is there a safe way?" they asked.

"Let me rephrase that. We are exploring Vegemite's neck because we think he has a focus of infection. We suspect the esophagus might be perforated, but we don't know for sure. Let's say we knew for sure there was an esophageal problem; a mass for instance. What approach would we use then?"

They thought about it for a moment, "Ventral midline."

"Exactly! If we go down the ventral midline we know we won't damage anything vital. We can separate the important structures and expose the trachea and esophagus. If they don't appear damaged, we can retract the carotid artery and work our way into the damaged musculature to debride and drain it."

In other words, let's go from *the known to the unknown.*

So we ended up incising relatively normal tissue, identifying the structures we would rather not damage, and were able to identify a normal looking espohagus, which we left alone, and a large area of muscular necrosis that we were able to debride and drain, then manage with a tie-over bandage (Figure 10.4B). Vegemite recovered uneventfully, with no neurological sequelae, and I was a convert.

The strategy of working from the known to the unknown is a useful technique for all surgical procedures, whether it be in the retropharynx, the abdomen, or the limb.

Can't find those tiny retained testicles? Find the ductus deferens and pull on it, then look or feel for movement in the inguinal fat pad. Can't locate the ureter? Put some gentle traction on the kidney and see what stretches. Or look for the small ureteral blood vessels traversing the retroperitoneum next to them. Can't find the adrenal? Look for the phrenico-abdominal vein.

This type of flexible thinking may also help you find your way when the satnav breaks down.

11

"It Will Be Interesting to See Whether That Works"

How to Be a Creative Surgeon

I was attempting to recreate the loaves and the fishes miracle by assigning our small group of surgery demonstrators to a much larger number of student teaching laboratories when I became aware of our lead tech, Gigi, standing behind me. Ever polite, Gigi rarely interrupted me when I was occupied. According to the urgency of the situation, she would wait a variable amount of time then make her move.

"Ah, Dr. Hunt ..."

This morning, I was relieved to be liberated from a tiresome scheduling challenge, "Yep?"

"Flotsam is here."

Flotsam was a medium-sized, shaggy dog of dubious parentage, who was rescued by one of our administrative staff after being found floating in a storm water drain. Although ill-favored in the beauty stakes, she was a calm and affectionate dog who seemed genuinely grateful to have drifted into such a loving family.

"How's it looking?" I was referring to the surgical site from which we had removed a large perineal mast cell tumor five days earlier.

Gigi grimaced.

"Oh. Can you bring her back for me to look at?"

Gigi beckoned a student through the office door. Flotsam wagged along behind, dripping a trail of serosanguinous fluid.

The mast cell tumor had been located in an awkward position, lateral to the vulva and extending towards the pubis. The books were unhelpful regarding practical options for closing this area short of raising an axial pattern flap or sacrificing the dog's tail and, devoted as Flotsam's owner was, she could not afford major reconstructive surgery. So we'd done the best we could with primary excision, local undermining, and walking sutures.

A quick look at the site showed that a combination of tension and local movement was taking its not unexpected toll; a number of the original skin sutures were missing, and the wound was dehiscing.

"Shall we resuture it?" asked the student.

I don't mind resuturing if the original repair breaks down as a result of patient trauma or poor technique, but my simplistic view is that a wound usually starts to dehisce because there is a problem with healing, and the sutures fall out as a consequence, rather than the reverse.

"It's the wound's way of telling us it needs to heal by second intention," I tell my students or, in the case of the client, "It wants to heal from the inside out."

Flotsam's wound was under tension, there was constant motion between her legs, and who knew what local factors were at play subsequent to the mast cell tumor.

Unwelcome as the idea was, I felt we were better to leave Flotsam to heal naturally.

"We'll manage it as an open wound while it granulates and contracts. There's no doubt it can heal, it will just take some time."

I wondered about that wisdom a few days later, when the wound separated completely and we struggled to keep a bandage in place for more than a couple of hours. I finally thought

Pitfalls in Veterinary Surgery, First Edition. Edited by Geraldine B. Hunt.
© 2017 John Wiley & Sons, Inc. Published 2017 by John Wiley & Sons, Inc.

that we might be better not to bandage the wound at all, but it was a tough call when Flotsam was urinating almost directly into it.

If only there had been a superior option for surgical closure in the first place!

Thanks to a fortunate combination of assiduous owner and extremely tractable patient, Flotsam's wound contracted to a barely noticeable furrow in the six weeks before Mamushka arrived.

Mamushka, a six-year-old Cairn Terrier, was led into the consulting room by her human, Eddie, who was exactly the same age; Mamushka and Eddie were accompanied by their mother, Tara.

"Mamushka," Eddie announced. "Has a problem with her tushie."

I read the file before they arrived. Their local vet did a marginal excision on a mass from the perineum about two weeks previously. Although the wound healed normally, histopathology confirmed the mass to be a mast cell tumor; incompletely excised. Mamushka was here for re-excision with wider margins.

"Show the doctor your tushie," Eddie instructed his fur-sister.

My heart sank; it was Flotsam all over again. The wound was located a centimeter lateral to the vulva, extending down to the pubic area. Even if I re-excised it with a 2-cm margin, I would struggle to close the wound at all, with a very high likelihood of dehiscence. Undermining would provide minimal assistance, and there was no local source of loose skin for an advancement flap or an H-plasty. I had closed similar wounds in male dogs by recruiting skin from the scrotum, but Mamushka had too many X chromosomes.

I chatted with Tara about the pros and cons of surgery and the potential for wound dehiscence. She had already decided that surgery was the best option for Mamushka, even if it meant multiple visits for open wound management.

"Mamushka needs to have surgery," she explained to Eddie, who nodded calmly.

Tara signed the forms and the student took Mamushka's leash.

Eddie's calm demeanor vanished. "No!"

"But she has to go into hospital," his mother explained.

"I want to go with her!"

With an admirable balance of compassion and determination, Tara persuaded Eddie to let his best friend go. As the dog was led from the room, huge tears spilled from his eyes and while his mother coaxed him back to reception we heard his heart-rending cries, "Mamushka, Mamushka, Mamushka …"

We took the dog to our surgery office to finalize the surgical plan. Eddie's cries cemented my desire find a better strategy than the one we used on Flotsam; but what?

I had them hold Mamushka while I palpated the skin around the proposed surgery site, working out the lines of tension and whether the local skin was mobile or stretchy. Then I stared quietly at the site and put my mind to work.

I reflected on what I had read or heard about mast cell tumors near the vulva. Four months previously, I had been in Newcastle, UK, giving a joint presentation on wound management with Ronan Doyle, an English surgeon. Ronan talked about how he liked to "scrunch" the skin around the surgical site to evaluate its usefulness for reconstruction. Ronan had also presented a case with a mast cell tumor on the vulva itself. Although it seemed to present a major reconstructive dilemma, the solution was simple: the vulval fold itself acted as the surgical margin. I studied Mamushka's vulva; if only her mast cell tumor had been in a slightly different location. Asking the student to hold Mamushka still, I gently pulled her vulva aside to see the surgical scar better.

"It's a shame," I said, as the elastic skin stretched between my fingers, "she's got this great vulval fold she doesn't need!"

When deciding how much skin to remove during a routine episioplasty for vulval fold dermatitis, I usually incise around the mucocutaneous junction of the dorsal commissure, undermine the vulval skin, and then pull it ventrally to cover the vulva itself (Figure 11.1A). Students and surgeon alike marvel at the large

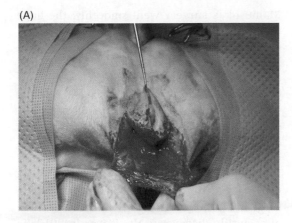

(A)

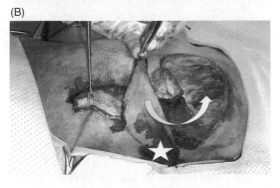

(B)

Figure 11.1 (A) Demonstrating the extent of the vulval fold resected during an episioplasty performed with the patient in dorsal recumbency. (B) Creating the vulval fold flap to close a perineal defect in a female dog (dorsal recumbency). The incision is following a line drawn along the dorsal and ventral aspects of the vulval fold with the base of the flap to the right (white star). Before completing the incision, the surgeon is checking the mobility of the skin flap and the tension created by drawing the donor site together. The surgeon is grasping the subcutaneous tissue with a skin hook and thumb forceps to avoid damaging the skin edges.

veil thus created. With the skin under moderate tension, I use a surgical pen to mark the line along which the mobilized skin overlaps the initial incision. Then I divide the vulval fold along that incision line, and thus allow the resulting two skin edges to be sutured together. This impressive flap of skin is then thrown in the trash.

All that lovely skin, I thought again. *What a waste.*

I scrutinized Mamushka's back end; frowning as the kernel of an idea sprouted and then sent down roots.

Why couldn't we use the vulval fold skin as a flap?

Any lecture or textbook chapter on creation of local skin flaps will emphasize that the success of a flap depends on its blood supply. Unless you are lucky enough to incorporate a direct cutaneous artery (in which case you create an axial pattern flap), local flaps require a wide enough pedicle to be adequately perfused by means of the subdermal plexus. Experiences with episioplasty had taught me that the perineal skin was richly vascular. Why couldn't we perform a partial episiplasty, but leave one of the lateral attachments to the vulval fold intact, enabling a vascularized flap of skin to be elevated and rotated into a defect next to the vulva?

Bingo!

I smiled at the resident who was in charge of Mamushka's case.

"I think I've worked it out." And so the vulval fold flap was born (Figure 11.1B).

I hate doing the same thing over and over. A curious dilemma seeing that – at least in surgery – everyone knows that is exactly what's required to become proficient. It probably explains my love–hate relationship with surgery teaching laboratories. They are an integral part of veterinary training, and the look of joy on a student's face when they finally work out how to bury a knot makes it all worthwhile. But it is a scenario where you have to choose a technique and stick religiously to it; the last thing students need before they have mastered anything is someone saying, "Well that's one way to do it, but here is another way you could try."

No, you need to choose a single technique, break it down to its simplest components, and help them to understand the basics before they encounter the nuances of how one might do it differently. Unfortunately, for many vets, that becomes the only way they will ever do it because that was how they were trained.

Going into practice, I was so terrified of making a mistake, even if I followed the textbook letter by letter, I was hardly inclined to branch out and make up my own way of doing things. And as we become more and more familiar with a technique, and better and faster at doing it, and we have achieved some success with our patients, the less likely we are to entertain new ideas. How many times have you heard one of your colleagues arguing black and blue that their way is the best, and justifying it with loose science and subjective observation? Luckily, we are moving towards a more evidence-based approach to help us choose between available treatment options. The problem is that someone has to come up with the various alternatives in order for us to have that choice, and that requires creativity.

My surgery supervisor had a habit of standing behind his residents when they stretched the apron strings and began to make their own decisions. His favorite comment was, "It will be interesting to see if that works."

It could – as you might imagine – be intimidating; especially as we floundered through the sweating stage of a surgery. Or – in good Australian fashion – it might be taken as a challenge; assuming we actually did know what we were doing at the time. Although my professor's comment seemed judgmental when I was a resident, I now think it was purely a statement of fact.

Yes, it would be interesting to see whether that worked.

Because if that did work, we had a new option.

I loved those early days, when so much remained to be discovered, and there was so little evidence for different techniques you could choose your own path with little fear of repercussion. We designed new skin flaps, and procedures for treating congenital heart disease and liver shunts. We trialled drug combinations, surgical implants, and medical devices. You might think, after that great flurry of activity, and following the exponential rise in surgical books and papers, there is nothing left to discover. What potential is there to be creative in your day-to-day practice when everything must be based on published evidence?

Think again.

Mamushka's surgery went smoothly: the huge flap from her vulval fold fit perfectly into the excision site allowing tension-free closure and a healthy respect for the subdermal blood supply (Figure 11.1B). It healed completely and without complications, ensuring that Mamushka was separated from her human soul mate just once. Two weeks after the recut her sutures came out and she was sent home cancer-free. It was a triumph![1]

When did this happen? In 1990, as I was starting out in my career as a soft tissue surgeon? In 2000, during my mid-career flush of scientific discovery? No, it was in 2010, as I coasted on two decades of experience. I wish I had thought about it in 1990, or 2000, but it took a series of seemingly unconnected cases to plant that seed that finally germinated when fertilized by the coalition of Mamushka's awkward wound, her sweet young owner, and my feeling of responsibility to help to find a solution.

I wrote Mamushka into a lecture for practicing veterinarians called "Wounds that Defy Closure," and have been asked to give it at virtually every Continuing Education event I have attended since. These are not cases where you can look up the textbook. These are the patients where there is not yet a published solution, or where the available options are too expensive, impractical, or just not acceptable to the owners: it is near impossible to keep a bandage on, the dog won't allow regular bandage changes, or the owners just can't afford it. These are the cases where you struggle to find an answer, but the buck stops with you. These are the cases that can torment you, where you cannot help but care, but if you find a creative solution it will be a highlight of your career.

To be creative is not to cast a net around randomly and hope to catch something worth keeping. It means thinking flexibly, using old

---

1 Hunt GB, Winson O, Fuller MC, Kim JY. Pilot study of the suitability of dorsal vulval skin as a transposition flap: vascular anatomic study and clinical application. *Veterinary Surgery* 2013; 42(5): 523–528.

technology for new purposes, trying different ways of getting past an obstacle: if you can't go through it, maybe you can go around, or over, or under. And simply because there is no published surgical approach for a certain condition doesn't mean it can't be done.

Vincent was an eight-year-old Labrador who presented for "old Labrador disease": not as playful, reduced exercise tolerance, a little arthritic in the back end, panting a lot. His appetite, of course, was fine.

He didn't have laryngeal stridor, so we ruled out laryngeal paralysis, which left many other options. The owner's main concern was the pear-shaped lipoma on his left dorsal abdomen, just behind his rib cage, but my resident argued effectively that it was hard to attribute Vincent's general unwellness to a lipoma.

We, and Vincent, were fortunate that his owner agreed to a minimum database. We weren't expecting much but when the thoracic X-ray flashed up we were forced to take the owner's concerns more seriously. The pear-shaped lipoma on Vincent's side was the crown of an entire fruit bowl. The fatty monstrosity had pushed its way between his abdominal muscles and rib cage, shouldered his left kidney aside, peeled diaphragmatic crus from epaxial muscles, created an uninterrupted highway of lard from skin to caudal vena cava, and was slowly moving towards Vincent's heart (Figure 11.2A).

On the bright side, Vincent's lipoma had done all the surgical dissection, leaving me the rewarding task of gently freeing its flimsy attachments in order to lift it out (Figure 11.2B). It left a massive hole, exposing a meticulous anatomic prosection of his epaxial musculature, his abdominal and thoracic cavities, the great vessels linking the two, and an adrenal gland that dangled rather aimlessly. I wished I could show this to our students as they struggled with first year anatomy.

Because the tumor had separated critical muscular structures, rather than destroying them, it was also straightforward to reappose them and thus close the impressive defect.

(A)

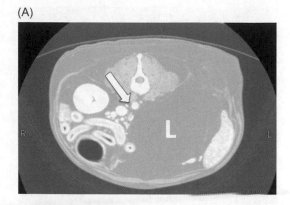

(B)

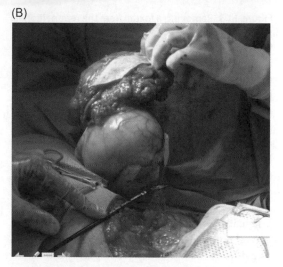

Figure 11.2 (A) Transverse CT image of a large lipoma (L) dissecting through the body wall to the retroperitoneum in a dog. The white arrow points to the aorta. (B) External (with attached skin) and internal components of the lipoma in (A). Removal of this lipoma provided excellent surgical exposure of the diaphragm and retroperitoneal structures. Courtesy of the Veterinary Medical Teaching Hospital, School of Veterinary Medicine, UC Davis.

When we finished, it looked as if nothing had happened!

I did nothing especially creative during Vincent's surgery, but I stored that anatomic vision for future reference. If the tumor could so neatly dissect the complex structures making up Vincent's mid-section, all the way to his very core, why could I not do the same? I was later delighted to read Staiger's paper – based on some

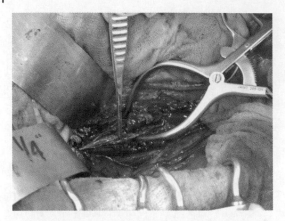

Figure 11.3 Removing a foxtail from the retroperitoneal space of a dog using the same approach for surgical exposure as in Figure 11.2.

excellent creative thinking – that described a single paracostal incision for accessing the cisterna chyli and thoracic duct.[2] Although I did not use the "Staiger/Vincent" approach for cisterna chyli ablation until much later, I did employ it successfully to find a grass awn that had migrated along the mediastinum and caused an abscess dorsomedial to the right adrenal gland (Figure 11.3).

You can be creative without being negligent; you can build creative solutions on a foundation of evidence-based practice. Expand your existing knowledge and experience to the novel situation. Use first principles and think about what you want to achieve; clarify your goals rather than knee-jerking from one page of the textbook to the next.

In the year I completed my Surgery Residency I was appointed to the University of Sydney as a lecturer in Equine Anatomy. I liked horses and by this stage my partner and I had accumulated three. But I had long ago given up the idea of becoming a horse vet, so my decision to take the job was mainly to acquire experience with

2 Staiger, BA, Stanley BJ, McAnulty JF. Single paracostal approach to thoracic duct and cisterna chili: experimental study and case series. *Veterinary Surgery* 2011; 40: 786–794.

university teaching, and see how things might morph from there. In addition to my responsibilities for equine anatomy lectures and labs, I demonstrated in canine anatomy labs; put my hand up to teach cardiovascular anatomy and embryology as I had developed a strong interest in cardiac disease during my PhD; and eventually took over canine neuroanatomy.

Becoming an anatomist was one of the best things that happened to me as a surgeon, as it led to an excellent understanding of how the body was put together and, consequently, how to take it apart safely.

I had no teaching responsibilities between semesters, so I was also appointed as a visiting surgical specialist to the university teaching hospital, where I spent most of my free time.

I was in the finishing stages of a total ear canal ablation when the operating room tech opened the door.

"We've got a ref vet on the phone. They need some urgent advice."

Leaving the student to place the final cruciate suture under the supervision of our anesthetist, I scrubbed out and picked up the phone in the sterilizing room.

"Geraldine Hunt speaking. How can I help?"

"Hi, thanks for coming out of surgery!" His relief was audible. "I've got a case I really need to refer."

"Tell me about it."

"It's a middle-aged cat. Went out yesterday afternoon and they didn't find it again until this morning. Distended abdomen and bruising. They think it was probably hit by a car." His delivery was staccato and succinct. "Long story short; we tapped it and got urine, and then explored it to fix the bladder rupture …"

"And …?"

"The bladder's okay, but both ureters have been transected."

My heart sank; I had no experience with ureter surgery in cats. For some reason, we did not see ureteral calculi with the same frequency they were reported in the USA, and I had never learned microsurgery. I was freaking out, and really didn't want to tell this vet that I wasn't the right person for the job, but …

"I'm not sure I can do much to help," I said. "Oh ..."

All I could think was that the ureters needed to be repaired and in a cat that sounded like a nightmare and well beyond my expertise. Because silence suggests an absence of anything further to contribute, I spoke out loud as I thought through other options. "Maybe we can find someone who has an operating microscope and does have the surgical skills."

I knew of one specialist group who used an operating microscope regularly.

"You could try asking the ophthalmologists if they are prepared to have a go."

In retrospect, it was not one of my better ideas, and was received by the ophthalmologists with a predictable degree of enthusiasm. The cat's owners were having trouble coming to terms with the severity of the situation; the cat deteriorated and was euthanized while they were still trying to decide what to do; and I was left wondering whether we could have done anything different.

Nowdays, I am familiar with various options for this type of case. We can perform repairs and place stents. The ureters can be reimplanted into the apex of the bladder or, if the ureters are too short, the kidney mobilized and drawn caudally, or we can tube part of the bladder to bring it forward. If all that fails, we have the very clever alternative of the subcutaneous ureteral bypass system (SUB).[3]

Had I considered those palliative options back in 1993 when speaking with that referring veterinarian, I might have suggested that he close the abdomen and send the cat straight over; assuming the owners could make the decision and gather a suitable monetary deposit in very

short order. Then I would have started a race against time to source the required devices and have them delivered as quickly as possible, so we could do something definitive before the cat became unsalvageably uremic.

Unfortunately, even today, the majority of veterinarians in practice around the world do not have the means to easily diagnose – let alone treat – a cat with bilateral ureteral disease. And in the fortunate but rare event the owners entertain referral to a specialist center, perhaps after lengthy conference with the rest of the family, the issue of keeping the patient stable poses the same dilemma as it did 23 years ago.

Pixie was a rare male Calico cat fortunate enough to live on a beach near San Diego. Although confined to an apartment, he liked to sun himself on the deck, watch the daily parade of human exhibits along the esplanade, and perhaps daydream about romping through the enormous sandpit that was SoCal.

When Pixie lost interest in his own sandpit, followed by his food bowl, and then shunned his breezy ocean lookout in favor of the broom closet, his owners whisked him to the local emergency center. Blood work and an abdominal ultrasound later, he was diagnosed with bilateral hydronephrosis and free abdominal fluid, which was shortly thereafter proven to be urine.

The presumptive diagnosis was bilateral ureteral obstruction with leakage of urine from either the ureter or the kidney.

Apropos of Chapter 4 it was, not surprisingly, the Friday evening of a holiday weekend. Rightly or wrongly, the referring vet and the owners believed that Pixie's surgery could not be performed anywhere in Southern California until the following Tuesday.

They decided their only chance was to drive the nine hours to UC Davis. Based on his rapidly deteriorating blood work, however, they had no confidence that Pixie would survive the trip and arrive in a stable enough condition to withstand major surgery of indeterminate duration.

Pixie's vet gave some thought to the situation. It was a catch-22: Pixie needed the surgery right

3 Horowitz C, Berent A, Weisse C, Langston C, Bagley D. Predictors of outcome for cats with ureteral obstructions after interventional management using ureteral stents or a subcutaneous ureteral bypass system. *Journal of Feline Medicine and Surgery* 2013; 15: 1052–1062.

Kulendra E, Kulendra N, Halfacree Z. Management of bilateral ureteral trauma using ureteral stents and subsequent subcutaneous ureteral bypass devices in a cat. *Journal of Feline Medicine and Surgery* 2014; 16: 985–991.

now, but could not have it. So Pixie's vet did a commendable thing; she started to analyze exactly what Pixie's problems were:

Problem 1: bilateral ureteral obstruction.
Problem 2: uroabdomen.

Problems 1 and 2 were leading to problems 3 and 4: pain and azotemia, the cause of Pixie's main clinical signs.

Then she thought about the exact reason each problem was impacting the cat (i.e., what was actually going to kill Pixie in the near future?)

Bilateral ureteral obstruction results in urine not being excreted normally.

Uroabdomen results in urine being reabsorbed.

Apart from providing pain relief, and short of fixing the ureteral obstructions, what could she do to minimize the threat posed by Pixie's underlying problems and stabilize him for his trip to Northern California?

Pixie arrived in our emergency room early on Saturday morning. He had been circling during the trip and when finally birthed from his travel carrier he was hog-tied by a tangle of IV lines.

"What the heck?" said the after-hours student as he disengaged each tube from its littermates, trying to work out what went where and – more interestingly – what came from where?

Pixie's vet had placed four lines: a right cephalic for intravenous fluids, a urethral catheter, a left nephrostomy catheter, and a closed-suction peritoneal drain. This would have been a good effort for our ICU, but for a vet in practice it was truly impressive (Figure 11.4).

Pixie's vet had rightly concluded that if something could be done to re-establish urine flow from even one kidney, and if absorption of the urine leaking into his peritoneal cavity could be minimized, then his condition should at least stabilize; if not improve.

The urine collection system attached to urethral catheter was sadly empty, but the nephrostomy bag contained a satisfying amount of serosanguinous fluid. And because Pixie was now able to excrete urine, it was safe to provide intravenous fluid without as much fear of over-hydration.

Disentangling the lines did more to help us understand what was attached to what than to improve Pixie's mobility, for he was suffering from the weird paralysis that afflicts cats with bandages around their midriff. However, he was capable of purring and miaowing, and seemed generally interested in life. He looked remarkably bright for four o'clock in the morning, and even more so for a cat suffering bilateral ureteral obstruction and uroabdomen.

Repeat blood work showed that his potassium and blood urea nitrogen (BUN) had improved during his journey from San Diego. Rather than being at death's door, and a high-risk anesthesia candidate, Pixie looked like a normal cat recovering after surgery.

Because Pixie's condition continued to improve over the next few hours, we decided to delay

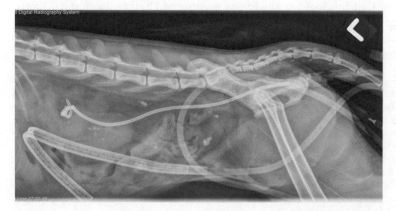

Figure 11.4 Lateral radiograph from a cat referred with bilateral ureteral obstruction and uroperitoneum. The referring veterinarian stabilized the cat by placing a nephrostomy tube (pig-tailed catheter), closed-suction peritoneal drain, and a urethral catheter. Courtesy of the Veterinary Medical Teaching Hospital, School of Veterinary Medicine, UC Davis.

surgery until he dropped down a couple of risk categories, and when we finally did operate to place bilateral SUBs, his uroabdomen had resolved and he breezed through the surgery.

So, why don't we do this with all our patients? Surely it is better to operate when they are stable, than unstable?

The first issue is patient welfare. Being in hospital is stressful for a cat at the best of times. A longer period of hospitalization with multiple catheters would amplify that enormously.

Another major issue is cost. This was no problem for Pixie's owners, but even one extra day of hospitalization is unacceptable for many clients, and the added expense of managing multiple tubes can be an absolute deal-breaker. Would it have been in Pixie's best interests to operate sooner? Possibly, if surgery had taken place immediately after diagnosis, close to home, and before his condition became too grave. Based on his likely risk category by the time he reached our surgical facility though, had he not been treated palliatively, his outcome might have been entirely different.

In veterinary practice we are always being challenged to find safer and more effective treatment options. We rise to that challenge, and with growing understanding of disease – coupled with emerging technologies – our potential has expanded rapidly. An additional challenge is to develop strategies that are cheaper and have less impact on the patient. It is far easier to come up with a treatment that is more costly, more complicated, and requires more advanced knowledge and equipment. But if we really want to make a difference to patient welfare worldwide, we have to develop solutions that are cheap, easy, and accessible to the majority of practicing vets and their patients.

The main thing I drew from Pixie's case was the power of working through a complex scenario, breaking it into component parts, and clarifying exactly what the goal is for each particular action. Pixie's vet didn't freak out and throw the cat into a carry cage for the car trip north. She thought logically, systematically, and creatively, and came up with a strategy that

probably saved Pixie's life. How might the outcome for the cat I saw so early in my career have been different had I not panicked because I could not perform the obvious definitive treatment, but if I had thought logically through the problem? I could have diverted urine and stabilized the cat in order to buy time for the owners to make their decision, and to investigate other options. Maybe at least one of the ureters could have been re-implanted? I never found out because I never tried, and I never tried because I felt forced into a snap decision. Systematic thinking allows us to buy the time we need to be creative, and can lead to an occasional miracle.

Our day-to-day cases do not usually require such complex treatment as Pixie, but they can be extremely challenging nonetheless.

Snitch was an 11-year-old Golden Retriever cross rushed into our practice following sudden collapse. Phil Collins could have beat out one of his famous riffs on the dog's abdomen, which would most appropriately have been titled, "Stomach Full of Air Tonight".

I was trained as a resident to operate on all dogs following an episode of gastric dilation, regardless of how easily they were decompressed, and whether or not the radiographs confirmed gastric torsion. Snitch was still alert, had no major underlying risk factors, and seemed a good candidate. His owners were reticent in light of his age, but they gave the go-ahead on the understanding I call them if I encountered anything that would adversely affect his prognosis. They cried when we discussed the possibility of euthanasia on the table; they didn't want Snitch to suffer unduly but they weren't yet ready to let him go.

"Let's take it one step at a time," I counseled.

The first thing I saw when I opened the abdomen was omentum covering Snitch's bloated stomach. He clearly had some degree of torsion. I ran the fingers of my right hand carefully down his left abdominal wall until I could feel the displaced pylorus. I used the flat of my left hand to guide the distended cardia back toward the left dorsal abdomen as I gently pulled the pylorus ventrally and to the right. The stomach rotated back to its normal position quite easily, but I was disturbed to see a large purple–red patch on the greater curvature. The short gastric vessels looked dark and thrombosed, with blood clots where some had torn. I had spoken with Snitch's owners about gastric necrosis and its uncertain prognosis, and their immediate response was that they did not want me to go ahead with stomach wall resection or any other heroic efforts. I would have to phone them and make them face their worst fear.

"Are you certain?" I imagined them asking.

"No, but it doesn't look good."

"But you don't know for sure?"

No, I did not; so I wasn't yet ready to make that phone call. But I knew I couldn't just go ahead and resect Snitch's abnormal gastric wall; his owners had been clear about that. It was more than just bruising or congestion; even when the surrounding stomach pinked up once blood began flowing more freely, this area looked dark and striated. On the bright side, it was not palpably thinner than the surrounding stomach wall. I pinched it but saw no contraction. I didn't like the way it looked, but I wasn't convinced that it was going to necrose. But if I left it, and it did perforate, I was condemning Snitch to days of discomfort as he suffered the inexorable outcome of septic peritonitis. So many "buts"!

I made a small incision through the serosa to see whether there was any perfusion and was rewarded with a very sluggish trickle of dark blood; better than nothing, but not nearly good enough. I knew I should phone the owners. Then my mind began to work. The stomach was traumatized and its blood flow was sluggish but I had seen other patients recover completely from bruised and congested bowel. I could suggest we wait and see. Had it been me, I suspect my surgeons might have opted for a period of abdominal drainage followed by strategic re-exploration, but we didn't have that luxury with Snitch for various reasons.

What were my main concerns with simply closing Snitch's abdomen and waiting?

First, I did not know whether the affected portion of his stomach would survive, especially once it filled with saliva and gas and the gastric wall tension rose, further compromising blood flow. Recurrent distention, or an episode of vomiting could tear it all apart.

Second, I would not know immediately if it was leaking, and he was developing septic peritonitis. I knew we would all feel terrible if things didn't go well and we just had to bide our time and wait for fate to declare itself.

What could I do to reduce the risk of not resecting the stomach and help me monitor the outcome?

Omentum would probably help; I often wrap it around gastrointestinal surgery sites, but it was unlikely to seal a large necrotic defect. I considered a serosal patch, but it was a very large amount of bowel to cover – I would be there all night! I could also invert the stomach and let it necrose into the gastric lumen, but that seemed an aggressive step if it had a chance to survive. In the end I opted for omentum.

After some deliberation, I also performed a pyloric antral tube gastropexy. This would allow me to keep Snitch's stomach completely decompressed, reduce the risk of vomiting, and maybe facilitate mural blood flow. I debated placing a Jackson–Pratt drain in his peritoneal cavity but decided against it; there was no evidence of leakage at the moment. I would monitor Snitch closely and if he showed the slightest indication of an issue, I could inject some water-soluble contrast agent into the gastrostomy tube and perform a gastrogram. If it leaked, we would have all the evidence we needed to recommend euthanasia. Armed with this strategy, I closed his abdomen and went to the telephone.

I spent the next three days imagining Snitch's discolored stomach wall, just as Dr. Meadows imagined the vulnerable triangle of her intestinal anastomosis, but I was not relying on divine intervention, I was banking on the stomach tube.

The reason Snitch stuck in my mind is that he made an almost completely uncomplicated recovery. I fasted him for 36 hours (a little longer than normal) and kept him on small frequent feeds of very moist food for a week afterwards. His gastrostomy tube yielded a lot of air and saliva initially, after which his gut sounds returned and the gastrostomy tube became redundant until it was pulled 10 days later.

I could have euthanized Snitch on the table, or I could have sutured him up and let the stomach take its chances, but the solution I chose gave us the best of both worlds and maybe it even tipped the balance. Who knows?

Mungus was a Golden Retriever who presented with a presumptive diagnosis of prostatic neoplasia. He had chronic urinary obstruction and had been catheterized numerous times over the previous few weeks. His bladder was the size of a rock melon and, despite posturing and straining, his dripping urine resembled a string of yellow pearls that could not quite coalesce into a stream. There was an ugly echogenic mass lurking within the bladder trigone, so things were not looking good. Without access to cystoscopy, we tried numerous ways to biopsy the site and thus confirm neoplasia, without success. The owner really wanted an answer before giving up on his best mate, so he elected for open exploration and resection, if possible.

The resemblance of Mungus' bladder to a melon was in no way diminished once I drained it in surgery. It was indurated and non-compliant, and although it could be deflated, it could not contract. Following weeks of distention and poor blood flow the detrusor muscle was scarred and indurated. It was hard to imagine – even if we relieved the urethral obstruction – that it could ever recover.

I located the sessile, cauliflower-like lesion at his bladder neck; this was surely a transitional cell carcinoma. It was beyond resection, creeping right up to the ureterovesicular junctions. But Mungus' owner still needed proof and asked me to biopsy it.

"He still won't be able to pee normally," I warned.

"Then put the tube in him." We had discussed urinary diversion to palliate Mungus' signs.

At the time of writing – 2016 – we would consider a stent for this dog with this owner, but how many other dogs are out there for whom a stent is not a viable option?

I could have placed a urethral catheter, but if you've ever had one yourself, you will know they are painful, and liable to be removed by your unimpressed patient. So Mungus got a cystotomy tube while we waited for his biopsy results.

Unexpectedly, histopathology revealed no evidence of cancer, but rather a florid inflammatory reaction. For want of something better, we diagnosed granulomatous urethritis.[4]

"I knew it!" said Mungus' owner, which impressed me as the condition had never been reported previously in a male dog. "How are you going to fix it?"

I could not fault his positive attitude.

"We can try an anti-inflammatory or corticosteroids, and see what happens."

One of the things I knew for sure was that Mungus would develop a urinary tract infection from his indwelling foreign body (i.e., the cystostomy tube). But if the eosinophilic mass shrunk, perhaps his poor scarred bladder might be capable of generating enough pressure to overcome the urethral resistance and reduce his dependency on artificial means of urination.

The owner read my mind. "How long before you can pull the tube out?"

Having seen his bladder, I was doubtful that Mungus would ever be able to pee on his own.

"I'm not sure," I said honestly. "It depends how effectively he can void."

A week later, Mungus' owner called to say he was urinating a weak stream. "Can we pull his tube out yet?"

"That depends on how much urine is left in his bladder."

Between us, Mungus' owner and I developed a strategy for monitoring his residual volume. Mungus would be allowed to urinate naturally, with his owner collecting the resultant liquid.

---

4 Moroff SD, Brown BA, Matthiesen DT, Scott RC. Infiltrative urethral disease in female dogs: 41 cases (1980–1987). *Journal of the American Veterinary Medical Association* 1991; 199: 247–251.

Then he would drain the bladder using the cystostomy tube and compare the volumes.

In the first week, Mungus struggled to pee out a quarter of his bladder volume. In the second week, he was managing half. Even though this was major progress, I warned the owner not to expect miracles. Mungus owner just smiled knowingly as he walked out the door.

Another two weeks later – over a month since surgery – Mungus' owner reported the dog was consistently able to pass 90% of the urine in his bladder.

"It's time," he said.

I asked him to bring Mungus in for one last measurement before the tube came out. We walked Mungus to the lawn outside the clinic.

"Mungus, NO!" said his owner as the dog cocked his leg on a wooden bench. Mungus dutifully lowered his leg and waited. His owner fished around in his backpack and pulled out a Royal Doulton teacup with a delicate floral motif. He squatted next to Mungus and held the teacup beneath the dog's prepuce. "Okay, buddy." Mungus let go and a torrent of urine ensued.

"Very nice, mate," said his owner, closely admiring the contents of the teacup to the horrified stare of another client walking her Pomeranian on the same lawn.

He flashed her a grin and she fled towards the parking lot.

"I get that a lot," he laughed as he emptied the slightly turbid, odiferous contents (Mungus did, indeed, have a refractory UTI) from the teacup into a plastic measuring jug similar to those you would find in any kitchen.

He then opened the three-way stopcock of the cystostomy tube, which dribbled a scant amount of urine into the teacup. His point proven, I relented and we pulled the cystostomy tube, to everybody's great relief. Mungus went on to live a happy life free of urethral obstruction and died at 13 when he ate the netting from a bag of oranges.

I have, ever since, been an ardent believer in the restorative power of decompression; but have preferred to drink my tea from a mug.

As I hope I have illustrated, the main theme of these various cases is that you can develop your own solutions, even when faced with a situation to which there is no discrete answer. Maybe you have experienced the "peek and shriek" phenomenon? You get into an exploratory and find something you (i) weren't expecting, (ii) don't recognize, or (iii) have no idea how to fix.

In Chapter 2, I suggested starting somewhere and seeing how things progressed. Let's say you have done that and made no progress, and now you are thinking about what to do next. Here is a checklist that might be helpful:

- Am I likely to refer this case? If so, take as many diagnostic samples as seem appropriate.
- Is the disease causing clinical signs that can be palliated in some way while the owners make decisions, or have time to say goodbye, or until another treatment option becomes available? I have given some examples earlier.
- Is there anything else I could be doing to facilitate future treatment? At the very least, try not to do anything that might complicate future treatment.
- Is it really as bad as I think, or does this patient just need support while things improve?

Don't be afraid to follow your instincts sometimes, even if they take you down a path you haven't trodden before. You can't always follow the pack and – who knows – you might just discover something nobody else has thought of!

12

When the Unthinkable Happens

Mishaps, Mis-steps, and Medical Errors

I love hanging out in Radiology.

It has a different pace to the rest of the hospital: lights are muted, people cluster around viewing screens – pointing and murmuring; things happen one at a time and at a civilized pace, and there is almost no banging or screaming. It is a great place to escape for a few minutes. And sooner or later, anything in the hospital that is half-way interesting – to a surgeon at least – passes before the X-ray beam.

It could just as easily have been a pharyngeal mass, or an intestinal foreign body, but this particular morning we were inspecting CT images of an intermuscular lipoma.

"99 red balloons, floating in the summer sky ..."

Heads turned at the surprise interruption and I sheepishly muted my cell phone. Our radiologist's voice followed me from the room. "Nice ringtone."

"Hello?"

"This is Marie, from reception. I have a vet on the phone. She's in the operating room and needs to speak to a surgeon urgently."

"Sure, put her through."

A moment's silence, then, "Dr. Hunt? Thanks for talking to me."

"No problem, how can I help?"

A rush of words. "I am operating on a cryptorchid dog and I just accidentally removed his prostate."

Whoa, I thought. *Not what I was expecting!*

She was in tears, "I feel terrible!"

What do you say to someone in that situation?

"The first thing it's important for you to know," I told her, "is that you're not the first vet this has happened to."

She stopped crying, "Really?"

"Really. Lots of people make mistakes."

And I should know, because I have made several.

Mistakes are not accidents, not surgical complications. Mistakes are when you do something deliberately, or choose not to do something, when you should have known better. When most vets under the same circumstances would reasonably have been expected to do it differently.

Scrotal swelling from edema or hematoma is an occasional complication of castration that can happen regardless of how well you perform the surgery.

A change in temperament, activity, and body-weight is an expected sequela.

Removing a dog's prostate when you were trying to remove a testicle is a mistake no matter which way you spin it.

Although – on paper – there seems a clear distinction between a mistake (or medical error), a complication of surgery, and an expected sequela to surgery, identifying the difference can be difficult in real life; especially in the eyes of the client. A mistake can also be because of an omission, rather than a discrete action. And despite our best efforts to turn medical errors into accidents in the eyes of those who might judge us, in the wee small hours of the morning, when our defenses are low, we can't fool ourselves.

Pitfalls in Veterinary Surgery, First Edition. Edited by Geraldine B. Hunt.
© 2017 John Wiley & Sons, Inc. Published 2017 by John Wiley & Sons, Inc.

Was it a mistake or an accident when I skewered the cat's aorta while pinning its lumbar vertebral fracture? I think it was an accident, but would it have happened in the hands of someone more experienced in that technique? Probably not.

Was it a mistake or an accident when I transected the dog's mesenteric artery while removing an adrenal tumor? I justified it as an accident on the basis that the adrenal mass was *surrounding* the artery, rather than displacing it as I expected. But if I had been watching more carefully, or had scrutinized the surgical anatomy more thoroughly when reviewing her CT, maybe I would have identified the problem before it became irreversible.

Was it a mistake or an accident when I held the telephone to my chest as I told a colleague, "I am just speaking to a difficult client," then returned to the phone to find anger had morphed to outrage when the incensed subject of my conversation spat, "so now I'm a *difficult client*!" Mistake or accident, it was one I took great pains to avoid a second time!

Bitsa was a seven-year-old spayed Kelpie cross. She presented for perineal irritation caused by a grape-sized mass in the vicinity of her left anal sac. Cytology showed inflammation, raising suspicions of an anal sac abscess. Despite a long course of antibiotics, the mass continued to grow and a punch biopsy suggested some form of sarcoma. Bitsa began having problems defecating and came to me for surgical debulking. I was ambivalent about surgery; the mass was locally invasive, poorly circumscribed, and would be impossible to remove with margins. If it really was a sarcoma, Bitsa's long-term prognosis was poor and who knew whether the surgical wound would even heal. But her owners were determined to buy her some time, so she was dropped off for surgery.

It was Friday, and the Friday night specials had come early, starting to mass the previous night and continuing through Friday morning. We ended up with nine cases on the board and, as they were all relatively uncomplicated, the surgery resident and I decided to "divide and conquer."

"I'll do Bitsa," I said. It was going to be a bloody and rather unrewarding surgery and I thought the resident might prefer to do the perineal urethrostomy.

It was early evening when Bitsa finally rolled into the operating room and was positioned in the perineal stand. I checked on the resident who had made excellent progress with his cat and was finishing the skin sutures.

"You get started on treatments," I said, "I'll take care of this one."

Left to my own devices with a student, I got through Bitsa's surgery in good time. The mass was firm and gristly, and quite hard to dissect around. I used electrocautery to peel it from the surrounding tissues and although there was a small puddle of blood on the floor at the end, the surgery site had minimal ongoing oozing. I had managed to prise the mass from the rectum and vagina without perforating them and, on balance, was happy.

"I warned the owners that this is going to recur," I told the student, "and we always worry about wound healing when we leave neoplastic tissue in the wound bed, so I'm not sure we have done a lot to help Bitsa, but hopefully we haven't done too much harm."

When Bitsa went home the following day her perineum and surgical wound looked remarkably clean and dry, with minimal swelling. Her owners phoned another day later, delighted that she had pooped normally for the first time in weeks.

Then I went on vacation.

I had been back about two hours when our surgery tech handed me the office phone and said that a referring vet wanted to speak to me.

"Hi, how's things?" I asked.

"I'm good, but Bitsa is having problems."

I wasn't surprised, but said, "I'm sorry to hear that."

"I'm not sure whether they told you, but she started having discharge from both her vulva and from the wound a few days after surgery. And it got progressively worse, so she came back for a recheck, and more antibiotics."

"That's bad news," I said. "I was worried about wound healing from the start, seeing as we couldn't get margins."

"Oh, the histopath came back as inflammation."

"Inflammation! Really?"

The vet continued, "Anyway, the owners just phoned tell me that ..."

The wound had dehisced, I predicted mentally.

" ... they pulled two gauze sponges from her vulva this morning".

Shit.

"My goodness!"

"Yes!"

I was teetering on that ledge of hope to which you cling before the gravity of realization takes you down. "What sort of sponges?"

"Surgical sponges."

My tenuous hold broke and I dropped off. "Oh ..."

In the days that followed, I spent a lot of time wondering how this had happened. The owners came in for a meeting and brought the offending sponges with them. Any last hope that the gauze might have come from another source dissipated when I saw the same radio-opaque strip used in our surgery packs. Although Bitsa had undergone one previous surgical exploration at another practice, I could only conclude that these sponges were ours. Or, to place responsibility where it was due, they were *mine.*

The surgical dissection had created a large hole, and I knew I had packed it with gauze while I managed the bleeding. But I was sure I lavaged the wound thoroughly before closing it. Because we were working outside a body cavity, though, we had not performed a sponge count, so I really had no idea whether they were all accounted for.

It was not until some months later – lying half awake in bed one night – I remembered what had happened. As I dissected around the mass, I lost track of its relation to the vaginal wall. I packed the vagina with gauze in order the palpate it more easily as thus avoid any perforation. I had clearly forgotten to take them out again.

The only bright note was that, relieved of her vaginal gossypiboma (retained surgical sponge), Bitsa healed uneventfully. And because her mass was inflammatory, rather than neoplastic, the surgical excision removed enough tissue to reverse the process and her perineum returned to normal. There were many more events between that telephone call from the referring vet and Bitsa returning for her final recheck, and we will explore those concepts later.

It is hard to write this chapter; nobody likes to see their mistakes hung out to dry. We want to represent our profession in a way that showcases our dedication, compassion, and efforts to provide the best quality of care. We don't want people thinking that we are callous, careless, or downright negligent. You rarely see a textbook chapter dealing with errors. But this book is about those things you don't get from the textbook; the hard-learned knowledge that comes from getting out there and doing it for over 30 years.

One of the major things this profession taught me was that mistakes will happen. When I struggled for some way to reassure the vet who had just performed an inadvertent prostatectomy, I was not excusing her. I wasn't trying to make it "okay." Making a mistake like that is not "okay." It was a devastating error that had a significant impact on that dog's life. But mistakes are a fact of life, and sooner or later we each have to work out a strategy to deal with them, and to reduce the risk they will happen again.

Being a teacher also helped me to realize that, traumatic as it is, people can learn from my mistakes. Practicing in a university environment for most of my career, I have developed robust cutaneous hypertrophy. How to describe the emotional impact of overhearing two students describing the postmortem results from one of my surgical failures? Imagine that hollow feeling when your plane drops into an air pocket. And afterwards – well, it depends whether the postmortem confirmed your skills in the face of a terminal disease, or discovered a surgical error – in which case the turbulence can persist for a very long time. It is far less grueling to learn from someone else's mistakes than from your own. So, although it is hard for me to relive these moments, I consider myself lucky to be able to share them, so you might avoid those same traps.

It was Wednesday – just over a week before the end of the school year – and the clinic was humming. Surgery exams were being graded, and we were tying up as many loose ends as possible before we went to emergency hours for the holidays. I had one thing in my sights; a glorious 10-day vacation during which I would turn the phone off, sleep in, watch movies, lie on the beach, and generally recharge batteries that were one cup of coffee away from being totally flat. It was a reward after months of sustained activity in clinics, the classroom, and the laboratory. And it was almost over …

Rory was a 10-year-old male neutered Beagle who presented for evaluation of an uncharacterized left nasal mass causing him to sneeze out foul-smelling clots of blood-stained pus. His owner, Paul Wallace, was a professional triathlete with a strong interest in ocean swimming. I was also on the ocean swimming circuit – albeit in a very different class – but Paul was sociable and pleasant to the eye, and with the prospect of some R&R just around the corner I was feeling generous with my time; so we traded swimming stories.

Eventually it was time to admit Rory into hospital. His nasal mass had all the radiographic hallmarks of neoplasia but repeated blind biopsies had yielded only inflammatory cells.

"I think cancer is the most likely thing," I told Paul, "but there could be an underlying foreign body, or some other inflammatory condition."

We agreed I would surgically explore Rory's nose and see what I found.

"I'll be going in through the mouth," I said. I was a great fan of David Holmberg's ventral approach to the nasal cavity and had used it many times.[1] I debated leaving the surgery until after the holidays, but Rory's clinical signs were uncomfortable for him and vexing for his owner and – hey – this was a surgery I could do standing on my head!

Paul signed the consent form, which included the risk of complications such as bleeding, oronasal fistula, and failure to cure his disease. He paid a deposit at the front desk, and left for afternoon training.

The following day, we anesthetized Rory and prepped his mouth for the ventral rhinotomy. It was a "textbook" surgery; I got great exposure of the nasal cavity and it proved full of a similar substance to that with which Rory had been annointing his owner's apartment. I was a little perplexed to find no discrete mass, and disappointed there was no foreign body, but noses can be misleading like that. It can be hard to differentiate blood clots and pus from soft tissue. I biopsied the turbinates, lavaged the nasal cavity thoroughly, and packed it with gauze to reduce postoperative bleeding. Dogs tended to recover very quickly from ventral rhinotomies, so I anticipated that I would pull the gauze tape from the nostril tomorrow morning, and send Rory home by the end of the week.

As soon as I tied the continuous polydioxanone suture in the roof of Rory's mouth, I reminded Anesthesia about the packing in his pharynx and darted off to my office to grade surgery exams.

These were the days before online exam submission, and the papers sat waiting on my desk like a loose-leaf recreation of the continental divide; currently dividing me from my much anticipated holiday. For two hours I attempted to forge a path to the summit then I took a break to visit the recovery ward and see how Rory was faring.

He was sitting up in his cage; very awake. Because I made the approach through the mouth I had not clipped any hair from his head and apart from the tail of gauze protruding from his nostril, it seemed nothing had happened to him. I loved that surgery! I noticed the biopsy samples, in a labeled jar of formalin next to his cage; the student had not found time to submit them to pathology just yet. I pulled a form from the pigeonhole on the wall (no mechanism for online submission yet, either). I attached a sticker, wrote in Rory's details and began to fill

---

1 Holmberg DL, Fries C, Cockshutt J, Van Pelt D. Ventral rhinotomy in the dog and cat. *Veterinary Surgery* 1989; 18: 446–449.

out the "clinical signs" section: *mucopurulent discharge and blood from left nostril ...* when a switch tripped in my brain and I glanced at Rory.

I was sure the owner told me the discharge was coming from the *left* nostril. I checked the referral letter.

Yep; left nostril.

I turned to Rory again: the gauze tape was protruding from his *right* nostril.

How could that be? Had he somehow inhaled it and sneezed it back out the other side? Had the anesthetist left some gauze in the back of his throat and this was what I was seeing?

I looked more closely; the tape was attached to his right nares with a tiny drop of superglue. No mistake there.

I was lost for an explanation. I had operated on the correct side. I clearly remembered that exploring the nasal cavity to the left of his septum. Except ...

Except Rory had been lying on his *back* (Figure 12.1).

So much for this being a surgery I could do standing on my head. In fact, I wished I *had* been standing on my head; for then I might have been able to tell left from right.

The floor seemed about to collapse beneath my feet as I put the biopsy specimen back on the

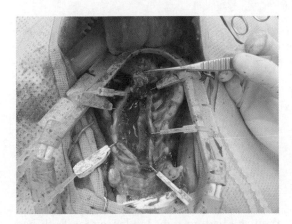

Figure 12.1 Ventral rhinotomy in a dog with nasal adenocarcinoma. Don't make my mistake by getting your left and right confused when your patient is on its back!

shelf, walked from the recovery room, dragged myself up the stairs, and sank into my office chair.

Ten minutes later, I composed myself enough to pick up the phone.

"Mr. Wallace, it's Geraldine Hunt, Rory's surgeon."

"Hi there! How's the old chap doing?"

"He's come through the surgery really well and he's up and asking to go for a walk."

"That's great news! I've been worried about him."

I steeled myself. "Mr. Wallace, I have to tell you something about the surgery. It ..." I didn't know what to say, but it came out, "It didn't go as well as I had hoped. I have to tell you ... I operated on the wrong side."

I expected an explosion; what I got was a moment's silence and then, "Oh my God."

"I am really sorry. It is my fault completely."

I realize many people consider this exactly the wrong thing to say; to so clearly admit my mistake. You will have to use your own judgment if you ever find yourself in this situation.

"The main thing I want you to know," I continued, "is that nothing I have done would interfere with Rory having the same surgery on the correct side. I know it means he has to have another surgery, and I know we don't want to put him through any more than absolutely necessary. But it would still be possible."

Paul Wallace was extraordinarily calm. "Well, I certainly appreciate your honesty." His next words were unexpected; a gift of which I felt very undeserving, "And I do understand that accidents sometimes happen."

Just as in Bitsa's case, there was a whole process to go through before Rory finished with us, and vice versa. Fortunately, neither patient died or suffered long-term discomfort as a result of my mistakes, but it could easily have been different.

Are these the only mistakes I made in my career? Almost certainly not. The trouble is, we don't always know we have made a mistake until much later, if at all.

Consider the cat that presents for inappetance and a large cystic mass where its left kidney

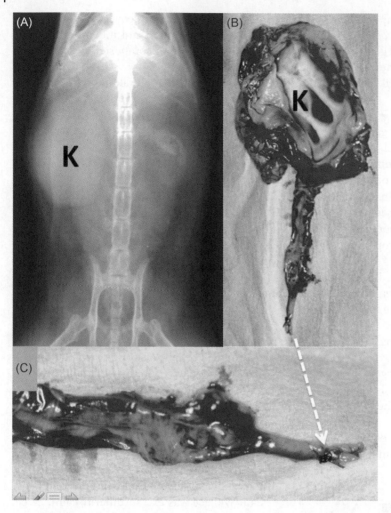

Figure 12.2 (A) Abdominal radiograph showing right-sided hydronephrosis (K) in a cat. (B,C) The hydronephrosis (K) was caused by ureteral ligation at the time of ovario-hysterectomy (arrow).

should be. It has advanced hydronephrosis, and the cause proves to be a surgical ligature placed five years previously when the cat was spayed (Figure 12.2). Alternatively, it may be a dog that presents for diarrhea and a palpable mid-abdominal mass. Sonography shows the mass to be poorly vascularized and not arising from anything in particular. The diagnosis: our unwelcome friend – the gossypiboma (Figure 12.3).

A couple of years ago, I operated on a ragged three-year-old bitch called Heinz. Heinz was a rescue dog and although supposedly spayed at the shelter prior to being rehomed, she kept showing signs of estrus. The owners weren't up for an ultrasound, so we opted to re-explore her on the strength of a presumptive diagnosis of ovarian remnant syndrome. She did, indeed, have an ovarian remnant; in fact, it was the entire left ovary. She had no right ovary, but then she had no right kidney, either. Both had been removed and the vessels secured within a single ligature. The shelter vet had achieved this complex resection through a tiny flank incision.

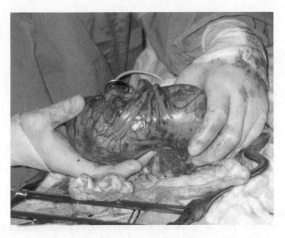

Figure 12.3 Long-standing gossypiboma in a patient with a mid-abdominal mass. Omentum has encased the retained surgical sponge.

I phoned the shelter manager and explained my findings.

"I am pretty sure that's not the outcome you and your shelter would like for your rescue pets," I said. She agreed, and said she would follow it up.

I hope she did, because much as we might dislike this sort of feedback about our patients, this is the type of mistake we need to know about, and soon enough to prevent it from happening again.

Is there a theme here? Are there any common threads between these various cases? I think so.

I doubt the vets who performed the inadvertent ligations and resections would have done so if they knew what was about to happen. They thought they were dealing with something else: a testicle instead of a prostate, an ovary instead of a kidney.

How could you make such a basic error? How can you ligate a ureter by accident? Having seen these things unfold in surgery practical classes using cadavers, I think our first major theme is poor visualization.

Do you have sufficient lighting, exposure, or retraction? Have you taken a moment to identify the structures entering and exiting an organ? The ductus deferens are a great clue when looking for a testicle, but remember the *opposite* end enters the prostate, so you need to use other clues as well. Ideally, you should be able to identify the ductus as it joins the epididymis. Even in a fat dog, it should be possible to mobilize an intra-abdominal testicle enough to identify its component parts. In short, if you can't positively identify it, *don't cut it out!* It's hard to know the real reason for accidental ligation of a single ureter as the cases often come in a long time after the offending surgery. But the ligatures are usually near the neck of the bladder and I suspect the ureter gets incorporated in a clamp when trying to secure a bleeding uterine artery.

The second major theme is busyness.

In both Bitsa's and Rory's cases, I was in a rush; I viewed their surgeries as simple procedures the likes of which had gone many times without a hitch. In both cases, there was a clearly identifiable moment at which the mistake could have either happened or not happened. If we had done a sponge count, I would not have forgotten the vaginal packing. If I had used the same system we use for anal purse string sutures, or tourniquets – to put a label on the dog's head that is only removed when the suture is removed – it would not have happened.

If I had taken a moment to check Rory's surgical positioning, maybe run through the procedure with my assistants before diving in, I would not have operated on the wrong side. I would never amputate a leg or resect an ear canal without double-checking that I was on the correct side. Why was Rory's nose any different? I was tired and distracted for both Rory's and Bitsa's surgeries, otherwise I would probably have remembered to do those things.

So our third major theme is fatigue.

And the final theme is absence of a "safety net."

I think of all the mistakes I "almost" made, but avoided because I, or someone working with me, remembered in the nick of time.

On the days I operated on Bitsa and Rory, I had no safety net. I might not have had my mind on the job, but nobody else was paying attention, either. They were certainly paying attention to their own responsibilities; we had no anesthetic problems in these patients, no equipment failures, no drug overdoses; so they did their own jobs immaculately well. And I am sure, had I asked them for help, they would have happily given it. But I did not even think to ask, and hence when I was about to make a mistake, there was no-one to step in.

I now know when I am entering what I call the "danger zone." When I am more likely to make a mistake. I am tired, stressed, overcommitted, rushing from one thing and one place to another. I can identify it and I know I must be extremely careful. It doesn't matter whether I am at work, or driving, traveling overseas, or even riding my bicycle. And I realize I can't do it alone. I can't be doing all those things *and* watching my back.

"I just want to let you know I have a lot on my mind at the moment," I tell the people working with me. "So please help me by double-checking, and if you are concerned about anything, if you think we've forgotten to do something we planned, or things aren't unfolding the way we discussed, please say something!"

In order for this to be effective, though, you must create an environment where people are willing to speak up. Surgeons can be intimidating at the best of times. How easy is it for a student, a technician, or even a resident, to tell their supervising surgeon they are about to make a mistake?

An even better way to create a safety net is to use checklists. The aviation industry worked that out a long time ago, and the medical profession more recently followed suit. But checklists only work if you identify all the critical components; then actually follow them.

Having a team of people to work with, ensuring everyone understands the goals and plans for a procedure, and everyone takes responsibility for its safe conclusion cannot be underestimated. Thank goodness for my surgical team who have saved many a day: the observant group of techs, students, clients, and peers who can point out the errors that are about to happen, the things I have forgotten, contribute ideas when I am fresh out, cheer me up by telling even more miserable stories of their own experiences, and share the delight when we occasionally pull off the seemingly impossible.

13

Things Went South – Now What?

Some surgeons never make a mistake.

They may have adverse sequelae but they do not have "complications." Some cases don't go according to plan but that is usually the fault of the technician, the owner, or even the patient.

"He had facial nerve paralysis afterwards, because the infection was so bad."

"He bent the pins in his tibial fracture, because he put too much weight on it."

"The wound got infected, because his owners let him lick it."

I envy these surgeons; they are not sentenced to a lifetime of questioning, wondering, even soul-searching. They sleep well at night and have an unshakeable belief in their own excellence. I wish I had their confidence, but I don't. I also think they might be deluding themselves.

Regardless of who is to blame for your poor surgical outcome, though, you do have to salvage the situation. After you've made that difficult phone call, or gone back to the consulting room to tell the owners about the badness under the bandage – what then?

I run through a scenario in surgery rounds. Sheba comes in with severe bandage disease after a mass removal and I ask the students to predict the owner's initial response. They come up with a range of ideas:

"How could this happen?"

"How could *you let* this happen."

"How much will it cost to fix?"

"Who is going to pay?"

These are all good suggestions but, regardless of what the owners might *say*, we conclude the concern uppermost in their mind is, "Will Sheena be okay?"

Having seen how small animal owners react to bad news – however skilfully delivered – I think this is the most critical thing for them to know; regardless of whether the adverse outcome results from a medical error or a surgical complication.

In the last chapter, I told you about the vet who accidentally removed a dog's prostate.

The first thing I told her was that she was not the first. My next words were, "This can be repaired. We have treated other patients with similar problems."

"Thank God!"

"There is a fairly high chance of some complication from the repair," I continued, "either urethral stricture, or incontinence, and quite possibly both. But we can place a stent if he develops a stricture, and we can use a urethral occluder if he becomes incontinent."

None of this focused on how much it would cost, who was going to pay, or the vet's legal position. Most critical was to work out a strategy to help this patient survive.

The strategy hinged on the vet's willingness to accept responsibility for organizing referral to a specialist for further evaluation. Following the principles I discussed in Chapter 8, she passed a balloon catheter retrogradely into the urethra and once it emerged from the transected pelvic urethra, she fed it through the proximal urethral stump and into the bladder. After the balloon was inflated it provided a mechanism for draining the

Pitfalls in Veterinary Surgery, First Edition. Edited by Geraldine B. Hunt.
© 2017 John Wiley & Sons, Inc. Published 2017 by John Wiley & Sons, Inc.

bladder of urine, and identifying the transected urethra when the time came for a definitive repair. I also suggested she tag the cut ends with non-absorbable sutures, tie them loosely, and leave them in situ when she closed the abdomen. Finally, to ensure the dog did not deteriorate and could be thoroughly evaluated and treated as semi-urgent – rather than a dire emergency – she placed a closed-suction drain in the caudal abdomen in the event that urine leaked around the balloon catheter. Now the dog was stable for transport to the local surgical specialist, and the vet could focus on talking to his owners.

When I met Bitsa's owners to discuss the retained surgical gauze, one of the first things I said was, "I am really sad Bitsa has had to go though this. We were trying to help, but instead we have injured her."

It is natural, when things go wrong, to focus on ourselves:

Am I going to be sued?

How much is this going to cost?

What will my peers and colleagues think?

These are all important questions. But right now, as I spoke with Bitsa's owner, I needed to demonstrate I cared more about their dog's welfare than my own feelings, and I would do whatever was required to find a way forward.

In the last chapter, I described my phone call to Rory's owner when I realized I had operated on the wrong side of his nose. After relaying the bad news, and receiving the owner's generous response that he "knew accidents did happen," I continued:

"My main concern right now is that Rory gets the treatment he needs, and that you are comfortable he is in the best hands."

The next part was difficult. "I realize you have no reason to trust me, so if you would prefer to see someone else, I can refer you to another surgical specialist."

Paul thought about this.

"No," he said finally. "I brought Rory to you because I was told you are a good surgeon, and you have been very straightforward with me. So I am comfortable leaving him with you."

I operated on the other side of Rory's nose the following day. The tissue I removed was subsequently diagnosed as an adenocarcinoma but – miraculously – the debulking procedure seemed to control the local disease (we did not have access to radiotherapy). Rory and Paul remained faithful clients until Rory died two years later from prostatic neoplasia.

I was fortunate, with Bitsa, that her problem had resolved itself and the wound was healing by the time I spoke to the owners. There was little doubt by then that the dog would make a complete recovery.

"*We very much appreciate the fact that Dr. Hunt took responsibility for the error.*" The owners wrote later. "*But we believe the hospital should cover the costs of Bitsa's treatment.*"

How our hospital responded is not the main point of this discussion. Every case is different, there often is no clear answer, and there are better-qualified people to comment on the legal and financial implications. What I *would* like to emphasize, though, is that veterinarians should develop a process for deciding on how to address such a request, and this should include your practice partners, hospital administration, and insurance providers where appropriate.

Despite my error in leaving the surgical sponges in her vagina, Bitsa's owners continued to use our hospital for several more years.

In large part, these benign outcomes from my surgical errors are probably due to the fact that both Rory and Bitsa were able to resume happy lives.

Sadly, I have seen other cases in which a clinical mistake – compounded by the way things were subsequently handled – led to animosity, mistrust, and threats of legal action.

So I have learned to respect the power of honesty, and our efforts to make the clients feel we really do care about them and their pet and we genuinely want to get the best result, even when things do not go as planned.

The next thing I hear clients ask is, "How will you make sure this doesn't happen again?"

I am proactive. I tell them we take every adverse event seriously. I let them know I will discuss it with at least one other clinician, to work out what we might do differently next time. If we are honest with ourselves, there is almost always something we might do differently next time, even if what we did was not, strictly speaking, *wrong.*

The faultless surgeons I mentioned at the beginning of the chapter never have to go through this process and – even if they do – they simply confirm their initial impression they did everything right.

If you want to gauge someone's level of self-reflection, ask, "What did you learn from this case?" and see how quickly they come up with a meaningful answer.

My mother suffered from pelvic osteonecrosis following radiation treatment. Her ischium fractured and did not heal well despite complex reconstructive surgery. I began to wonder whether her orthopedic surgeon really knew – or cared – what he was doing. One day, she returned from a recheck and said, "They are going to discuss me in rounds next week!"

Although I didn't know what that actually meant, or how many people might be in rounds, the mere idea her surgeon was going to talk to his colleagues made me feel better. One person might overlook some important detail, but surely a group were far less likely to let things slip through the cracks?

"I will discuss the case at our surgery service rounds," I told Rory's and Bitsa's owners, letting them know I was concerned enough about this mistake to put my ego aside and air it with my colleagues so we could all learn, and maybe change our protocols for the future.

"And I will use it as a teaching case for students and vets," I promised.

In Bitsa's and Rory's cases, I was clearly at fault; my error led to the adverse event. In other patients, I concluded that, should I see the same case again next week, I would act exactly the same way.

Which brings us to those cases in which a patient's undesirable outcome was interpreted as a medical error, even though the clinician was blameless.

Thor was a young Pit bull with a firm, painful swelling below his left ear. He was a strong, boisterous dog who deduced that the best way to make people leave him alone was to bare his prodigious canines and lunge. Needless to say, he was difficult to examine. The resident did a commendable job in that she not only examined the dog, but also obtained a FNA of the mass.

She came to me with the student and muzzled dog in tow, "He has a mast cell tumor."

In the limited time Thor allowed before he began spinning and foaming, I saw the mass had effaced the left side of his pharynx.

"I won't be able to get margins," I said sadly. "I'll be leaving macroscopic disease."

Thor was sent home with advice about non-surgical management, and medication to palliate his pain.

Two weeks letter, Client Services brought me a letter, "Can you comment on this?"

Distraught by Thor's rapid deterioration, his owners felt our interventions caused the disease to escalate; in particular, the "procedure" we performed had produced pain and a facial nerve deficit and Thor could no longer open his mouth properly.

"*None of this was apparent when we brought him in,*" they wrote. "*Your vets did some surgery that injured him while he was at the hospital.*"

I once had a young vet tell me, "It makes my blood boil when clients complain about our service!"

It annoys me, too, but if a client is concerned enough to complain it means something has really upset them – whether our fault or not – so it has to be taken seriously.

"They're clearly hurting," said Client Services.

I agreed they were hurting; it was a devastating diagnosis for any dog, let alone a robust young adult, but they were also blaming us and I had been asked to make a judgment.

"What surgery did we do?" As far as I knew, we discharged Thor with the advice that his mass was non-resectable.

"I think they are talking about the FNA."

My immediate thought was, *How ridiculous! A fine needle aspiration never hurt anyone!*

But that isn't strictly true. We aspirate things all the time, often with minimal thought or concern. Was it inconceivable that a sharp needle could cause nerve damage, especially in a strong young dog who was struggling at the time?

But why did the owners think we had done "surgery?" It occurred to me that if Thor had been taken to the treatment room for the FNA, and the owners had little medical knowledge, they might also have very little idea of what had happened to him back there.

In my early years as a veterinarian, a client wrote to the practice owner, demanding to know why I had taken her pet "out the back" for tests.

I spoke with her when she came in next. "I wanted to get a weight, and have the nurse hold him for us to collect blood."

She was clearly surprised. "You mean you have nurses back there?"

"Yes."

"I had no idea!" she exclaimed. "I didn't know what was behind those doors. I thought you were on your own and didn't want me to see how you held him down!"

Now you might think that any sensible person *should* know. But how would they? We take the day-to-day details of our practice for granted, because we know them so intimately, but it is wholly new for many of our clients.

Now, I try to introduce my clients to at least one other person who will be involved in their pet's care if they have to be taken "out the back," or admitted into hospital. I try to pair them with one of the techs so they feel they have a "friend behind the scenes." And if time permits, I organize a quick tour of the hospital so things are not left to their imagination.

I am going to digress for a moment and talk about the value of technicians. A good technician can be your greatest asset, and your best friend. Their qualifications and their pay scale might be tabulated, but their innate powers of observation, compassion, and ability to relate to clients and patients are unquantifiable. Their ability to detect trends and identify changes, their instincts about your patients, and their confidence in communicating with you are intangibles you will only appreciate after working closely together. Early in your career, you will learn a lot from your techs and receive invaluable support if you take the time to develop a good relationship. Later, even when you have more experience and think you know exactly what is happening with your patients, keep listening to your techs, for they are the ones with their finger on the pulse; taking Buster for a walk, watching how he moves, breaths, sleeps, eats, and does his natural business. They are the ones with their ear to the ground, in whom your clients will confide and who can tell you what they are thinking.

Concerns about Thor's owners' misunderstanding of how the hospital worked aside, their letter worried me. Could we prove the pain and nerve dysfunction was *not* caused by the FNA?

I could speak with the resident, but was hoping I would find the answer in the medical record; fortunately I did.

The consulting clinician had entered a comprehensive description of the initial examination, including: *Thor is presented for pain and swelling behind the jaw, and difficulty opening his mouth.*

In the notes on physical examination, I read: *Poor palpebral reflex and face droop, indicating facial nerve involvement.*

Thor was a very sad case, and we were not able to help him in any substantial way. We knew his owners were devastated by the news of his inoperable cancer. It felt brutal to respond to their letter, *Our medical records show that …,* but that was the reality.

If the initial consultation had not been written up comprehensively, or the resident had not performed a thorough physical examination and recorded the findings, things might have taken a very different turn.

So, my final piece of advice for all your patients, but especially those experiencing adverse events, is *keep good records.*

One of the excellent initiatives I saw at UC Davis was establishment of a Novel Procedures Committee. As centers for creation of knowledge, all university teaching hospitals regularly perform procedures that are either new or modified. If part of a clinical trial, they will have been approved by the local Ethics Committee, but plenty of cases fall between standard practice and clinical research. In Chapter 11 we explored how to be creative as a surgeon. The flip-side to creativity, though, is that you may be performing a procedure for the first time. And just how do you explain that to the client?

As a young vet, I felt very uncomfortable when a client asked, "How many of these have you done before?"

Because the answer was often one – or none.

During the early meetings of our novel procedures committee, we discussed just how to define the term. The concern was that "novel procedure" could potentially apply to any operation not previously been performed by that surgeon, for that indication, in that species.

This happens all the time in veterinary practice. Am I ethically or legally obliged to tell an owner that I am about to undertake a procedure for the first time on their pet? As so often the case, there is no cut and dried answer.

If there is solid published evidence for the efficacy of a certain procedure, and you have experience in other procedures in the same anatomic location, or using the same equipment, it would seem entirely discretionary.

If you have never applied a bone plate before, even if you are tackling a simple fracture, you should probably consider informing them.

I evaluate it on a case-by-case basis, and base my ethical position on my answers to the following questions:

"Would I want that information if *I* was the one having the procedure?"

"Will I feel uncomfortable if the owner asks me the question?"

No matter how my experience grows, I keep seeing things I haven't seen before. In my last week on clinic I operated on a dog with a urethral prolapse. In more than three decades of performing surgery, I had never carried out the procedure before. I had read about it, heard other surgeons discussing it, and looked at photographs. But although I knew what it entailed, I had never seen it myself. Was that something the clients needed to know?

If the clients knew, I asked myself, *how would they respond?*

I imagined that they might – quite naturally – ask whether the other surgeons had more experience? If so, they might ask that one of those surgeons operate on their pet.

Seeing as I have performed innumerable urethrotomies, urethrostomies, penile amputations, and hypospadias reconstructions, I decided not to discuss it with the clients. I did, however, ask one of my colleagues whether they knew of any tips or tricks. The procedure went smoothly and I felt comfortable that, were there to be a complication, I would feel I had given this patient the best available treatment.

You can see how this might raise a conflict of interest. We need experience with different techniques, but how can we get it if we hand cases we haven't done before to someone else?

Perhaps you can draw some conclusions from the examples above.

Should the owner ask, "How many of these have you done?" you might respond with, "My colleague has done several, and so I have asked her to be available so we can do the procedure together."

Sometimes things go pear-shaped through no fault of our own at all, but it still feels like a failure. Maybe we did not find something we were expecting: the dog with a palpable abdominal mass that has no macroscopic lesion when you open the abdomen; the cat with a radiographic bladder stone you can't find at cystotomy; the abscess that *must* have a foreign body inside of it.

None of us want to subject a patient to anesthesia and surgery when we end up doing nothing definitive; and justifying it to owners who then have to pay the bill can be even harder.

Millie was a West Highland White Terrier from the NSW Southern Highlands, which is the foxtail (or grass awn) capital of Australia.

She had a number of draining sinuses in her axilla; the tissue surrounding them was indurated and painful; the material draining from the sinuses was turbid and smelled bad. It repeatedly cultured positive for bacteria. She *had* to have a foxtail.

Unfortunately, two previous explorations failed to find the foxtail and Millie's owners were frustrated.

Reluctant to simply explore the area again, I suggested a fistulogram. We injected a water-soluble contrast agent through one of the larger sinuses. The network of tracts in Millie's axilla resembled a roentgenographic cauliflower.

Armed with this surgical roadmap, I explored the site again with the specific objective of opening a large cavity tracking along her lateral thoracic wall. I was rewarded by a rush of purulent material. I delved further, while students and techs watched expectantly, but the sinus terminated abruptly in a mess of granulation tissue.

Blast! It had looked so promising.

I took a step back and decided how to salvage the situation.

I imagined telling Millie's owners, "I didn't find the foxtail, but I was able to take a deep tissue culture."

I cut out a chunk of granulation tissue and dropped it into a culture tube.

I wasn't yet finished with our imaginary conversation, "And I also submitted it for histopathology, just in case she is reacting to some strange substance …"

This was a watershed moment in Millie's story, for histopathology showed that the "granulation tissue" was in reality a neoplastic lymph node.

Millie's procedure had morphed from failure to success, even though the final diagnosis was not a good one. Had I not taken the biopsy, not only would I have failed to find a foxtail, I would have failed to cure the dog – again – and the whole exercise would have yielded no diagnosis at all (Figure 13.1).

In Chapter 11 we glanced at the "peek and shriek" non-therapeutic procedure, and concluded

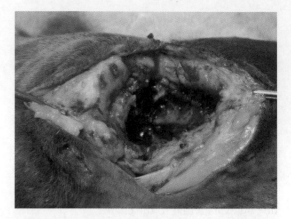

Figure 13.1 Surgical exploration of recurrent draining sinuses in a patient with a soft tissue sarcoma. No foreign bodies were found, and the diagnosis was made by deep tissue biopsy.

that taking diagnostic samples was an important step, along with some form of palliation if possible. The same thing applies to the "negative" procedure. Viewed through one lens, it could be seen as a failure. Through another, it is an opportunity to rule out some diagnoses, and take samples to test for others.

A word of caution though. If you are going to phone an owner and say, "Everything looked normal in there," make sure you have actually explored the region thoroughly.

Akela was a young adult German Shepherd who presented with fever of unknown origin and abdominal pain. Blood work suggested systemic inflammation. Urinalysis was normal. There was no radiographic evidence of discospondylitis. Chest radiographs were also normal. An abdominal ultrasound performed in the practice showed no major abnormalities, but was limited by gas in the stomach and colon. Based on Akela's pain on palpation of the abdomen, they decided to perform an exploratory laparotomy.

"They couldn't find anything abnormal," the owners reported when referred to me. "They think the problem is in deep – somewhere they can't get to."

Short of further imaging in the hands of a specialist, it seemed the referring vets had done a systematic job of evaluating this patient.

"Oh, and he is due to have his stitches out," they said.

We rolled Akela onto his back; the surgical incision spanned the middle third of his abdomen, from 5 cm caudal to the xiphoid to just behind his umbilicus.

Systematic as his vets had been in their work-up, I found it hard to believe they had been able to carefully explore the entire abdomen and, in particular, the dorsal abdomen, through this limited incision.

"We'll try another ultrasound," I said, then added a "white lie"; "We have a more powerful machine. We might be able to see deeper up towards his spine."

A short while later, we had our answer; there was a soft tissue mass near Akela's right kidney with a hyperechoic linear object in the middle of it.

I reopened Akela's abdomen the following day. In order to reach the paravertebral gutter in a deep-chested dog, my incision had to extend as cranially as possible; this meant starting right over the xiphoid process.

While demonstrating in anatomy labs, I learned the linea alba is not actually attached to the xiphisternum. If you extend a ventral midline celiotomy incision right over (ventral to) the xiphoid and between the deep pectoral muscles, you can separate the linea alba and caudal pectorals, leaving the xiphoid and its diaphragmatic attachments intact. What you need to avoid, when extending an incision cranially, is incising *lateral* to the xiphoid. You may cut the cranial abdominal artery (which bleeds!) and you also risk incising the attachment of the diaphragm and performing an inadvertent thoracotomy.

To test how easily you can incise over the xiphoid, make a celiotomy incision then run your finger, or a blunt instrument (Carmalt forceps for instance) between the linea alba and the xiphoid. You will find you can tunnel through the loose fatty fibrous tissue very easily.

Having started the incision cranially, I continued to Akela's prepuce. Had I been seriously concerned about his caudal abdomen or prostate, I would have extended it back to the pubis, but in his case I didn't think it necessary.

After placing the abdominal wall retractor, I performed a standard exploration of the abdominal contents. I was quickly greeted by the sharp end of a wooden skewer protruding from its coccoon of granulation tissue just lateral to the right kidney. The foreign body was on the move; migrating caudally along the right paravertebral gutter. I delivered it from the depths of the abdomen to a satisfying gasp from my assistants.

"Ah!" said Akela's owners, when I showed it to them. "We had kebabs at our housewarming party about a month ago! Thank you so much!"

When they came to pick Akela up after surgery, they gave me an expensive bottle of Cabernet Sauvignon.

As discussed in Chapter 3, if you can make a good case for exploration based on the available evidence, there is little wrong with performing an exploratory laparotomy even when no lesion is found. There is a problem when you explore a patient and *miss* the primary lesion. Especially if it is because you didn't follow good surgical principles.

I have no doubt Akela's primary veterinarian would have been the one to enjoy that rich, red wine had he made a surgical incision large enough to inspect the entire abdomen.

14

"There's Got to Be a Morning After"[1]

Things Went Wrong – Now Live With It

I looked around the silent room.

The students were avoiding one another's gaze, the resident's eyes were red. The techs busied themselves with paperwork. Nobody seemed to know what to say.

Matilda, the six-month-old kitten on whom we had worked around the clock following a dog attack, had just suffered a terminal cardiorespiratory arrest on the eve of being sent home.

The surgery team were in shock.

I felt the same: I loved that beautiful, cuddly, Calico kitten. We had congratulated ourselves on how well she was recovering, written a discharge statement in preparation for her release the next day, joked with the owners about how we hoped she had "learned her lesson" when it came to jumping the neighbor's fence.

Now we were making paw prints and sealing her in a black plastic bag.

"I should have run another blood gas," the resident said immediately after it happened.

The student asked, "Did I feed her too much this morning?"

It is always hard to lose a patient. If it is sudden, like Matilda, your feeling of satisfaction, your anticipation at seeing the smile on the owner's face when they are reunited, your general sense that you are making a difference evaporates, to be replaced by emptiness, regret, failure.

Even worse when you think it might have been your fault.

We had spent the better part of a week looking after Matilda. She dominated morning and evening rounds, the students teamed together and made up their own roster for monitoring, cleaning, and feeding and she won the hearts of everyone involved in her care. The first thing we did when we left the operating room after finishing another surgery would be to check in with the "Matilda shift" and see how she was doing.

She was our star patient and now, suddenly, she was gone.

Having faced this before, I counseled the downcast students. "We can't do anything more to help Matilda. But we can help the ones who are still alive."

It's a good strategy, as we have just as great a responsibility to all our other patients as we did to the one who died; but it is also a mistake to move on too quickly.

It's no accident that we make it into, and then through, veterinary school. We are high-achieving individuals with great commitment and focus. We work diligently, and expect to be successful. If we study effectively, we should pass the exams. If we do everything the instructor says, we should get full marks. If we work long hours, we should be valued employees. If we invest enough of ourselves, we should be repaid. If we try hard enough, surely we can be perfect?

Unfortunately, in clinics, it doesn't work that way. You can put your heart and soul into a case and still achieve a less than perfect result. You can lose the patient, or the client, or your confidence.

---

1 Maureen McGovern. "The Morning After" from *The Poseidon Adventure*, 1972.

Pitfalls in Veterinary Surgery, First Edition. Edited by Geraldine B. Hunt.
© 2017 John Wiley & Sons, Inc. Published 2017 by John Wiley & Sons, Inc.

None of us like to be criticized. Even worse is to be criticized in front of our friends. When our cases go badly, we worry about how it is going to appear to our colleagues and our clients. Are people going be mad at us? Are they going to think we are incompetent, stupid, or just plain culpable?

Harsh as the criticism we fear from those around us, I suspect the harshest criticism comes from within. Self-criticism is not objective, it's often not rational, and it is rarely fair. A certain amount of self-reflection is important, but when it moves beyond reflection to flagellation, it becomes a problem.

The most insidious thing about self-criticism is that it peaks when our defenses are low. The early hours of the morning can pass very slowly when we are silently beating ourselves up.

Putting a brave face on things, moving on from the patient we lost or the mistake we made and throwing ourselves into treatment of the living is a good way to get through the day. It is not necessarily a good way to get through the night.

For many years, I have been waiting for people to discover that I am really not that good at my job. I have rubbed shoulders with excellence in different veterinary schools, and wondered how I managed to fool my way into those hallowed halls. I always felt a whisker away from being revealed for what I really was: hard-working, nice enough to have around the place – hopefully – but secretly mediocre.

For a long time, I thought I was the only one to feel that way. Everyone else appeared so confident and capable. Surely they didn't lie awake wondering how long they could maintain the pretense? It wasn't until I listened to a talk by one of the other academics at UC Davis that I learned I was not alone. There is a name for this; they call it the "imposter syndrome."[2]

A recent internet search showed that imposter syndrome is alive and well in veterinarians, and there are many articles devoted to understanding and overcoming it.

Irrespective of whether we understand our inner imposter, all it takes is one really notable failure to shake our tenuous self-confidence. Even worse when it is a visible failure, and more devastating again when it leads to criticism from others.

Although, if you take a moment to think about it, when did one of your colleagues last criticize you? I mean *honestly* criticize you? Not a raised eyebrow, ambiguous comment, or silent omission that could be interpreted in any number of ways.

In fact, I don't think we criticize one another very much at all. I think we understand what it is like to be our colleague; how we struggle with cases, how hard it is to find the right answer, and how fickle biology can be.

So I suspect the root of my fear of negative feedback is that, in baring my actions for someone else to criticize, I also give myself carte blanche to cast stones. And it is the threat of that inner voice, nagging at me through the following days and nights, reminding me that my success was purely due to timing – and luck, and subterfuge – that really scares me.

In the past, I would do anything to avoid discussing difficult topics that might make me feel I had done the wrong thing. I set up defenses. There is an old saying, *the best defense is offense.* It is easy to be offended when someone suggests we are less than perfect. And because our colleagues are highly unlikely to criticize us to our faces, that dubious honor usually falls to our clients.

How dare Mrs. Bennett suggest I didn't communicate, or didn't treat Fluffy appropriately, or that I charged too much!

How dare she!

Self-righteous indignation goes a long way towards making us feel better about ourselves, and doubly so if we can share it with a friend. Our friend will surely agree with us, consolidating our position, and confirming the fact that

2 Clance PR, Imes SA. The imposter phenomenon in high achieving women: dynamics and therapeutic intervention. *Psychotherapy Theory, Research and Practice* 1978; 15(3): 241–247.

we acted honorably and competently – and that Mrs. Bennett is a witch!

The trouble with this approach, though, is that within the inconsiderate and inappropriate ranting of a demonic client, there may be a kernel of truth. Similarly, our inner imposter may be irrational and brutal, and unfair, but sometimes they also have a point.

How can we sift through the misconceptions, irrationalities, and general psychologic interference to identify those things that should be on our radar?

Intimidating as it might be, I have found the best thing is to seek a second opinion. It takes a while to work up to a real-life encounter, though, so I resort to my imagination. It is easy to be brave in your own mind and I am a surgeon, after all, so I start by tackling the issue head on.

"Did I do the wrong thing with Fluffy?" I ask myself.

My worse fear is a responding shake of the head, *"No. Dr. Bodgy struck again! How did you ever get a license, anyway?"*

An unlikely outcome. But then, *"Of course you did. You were perfect!"* is not very helpful. My inner imposter is not going to believe that for a second.

How, then, do I help my colleagues to give me some useful and objective feedback?

When my resident came to me after Matilda's untimely death and said, "I feel terrible!" I responded, "I'm sorry, it's tough feeling that way. What specifically is bothering you?"

She thought for a moment. "I am giving myself a really hard time because I should have done a blood gas before I put her in the wards."

The times I have spoken with colleagues and said, "I am giving myself a really hard time," they have sat up and listened. They have been understanding, thoughtful, and objective.

Sharing the problem makes it easier for me to deal with it.

Even better when, having shared my problem – the uncertainty about whether I did the right thing, or even the raw details of the mistake I made – we can move to an analysis of how it came about and, beyond that, strategies for avoiding a repeat.

"Okay," I said to my resident. "Let's talk through the sequence of events."

I didn't tell her not to worry, that she did everything okay, because I didn't know for sure. But I am not going to kick someone who is already kicking themselves by telling them that they should have been more careful. Rather, I hope that acknowledging the problem, and tackling it a piece at a time in the calm light of day, might help defuse those insidious doubts that come at night.

It takes courage to talk to another person about something that really scares you. And few things scare me more than feeling incompetent. But even if I have made a serious mistake, evaluating the circumstances leading up to it can help me realize that I did not make the mistake simply because I was stupid or inept, but because my processes, my checks and balances, my *safety net* let me down. And that gives me hope I might do better the next time around. In fact, I look forward to the next time, and being able to get it right.

In Matilda's case, I thought it a good idea to debrief the whole surgery team. It is not just the doctors who are hit hard by these events, it is our techs, our students, and the reception staff who check the patient into hospital and field phone calls from the owners.

We talked through what had happened during the course of that afternoon – our concerns, and whether we should have done anything differently. We don't know what killed Matilda. Her final set of blood results were normal, her owners were too distraught to contemplate a necropsy, and so we were left with the usual suspects: pulmonary thromboembolus, aspiration, underlying cardiac disease, and so on.

If we saw Matilda next week, we decided, we would not do anything differently. We went home saddened, but at peace with ourselves and the way we had looked after her.

Cathy Overall was sitting in Consult Room 3, crying. She had come in to talk about her Airedale, Miss McGee. We operated on Miss

McGee a week earlier to remove a thymoma associated with mild signs of myasthenia gravis. We all knew the surgery was risky. Cathy had signed a consent form containing a long list of potential complications. The surgery went smoothly. Miss McGee recovered quickly, and was sent home with a bill at the lower end of the estimate. It was all good.

Last night, though, Miss McGee returned to the emergency room with regurgitation, difficulty breathing, and muscle weakness. Rather than improving after surgery, it seemed her myasthenia was getting worse. She was rapidly heading towards the ventilator; an outcome that Cathy had already said was not financially feasible.

I opened the door and said gently, "I'm sorry about Miss McGee."

Despite the fact we made no mistakes, we informed Cathy of all the risks, and she did not blame us for anything, she sobbed something that made me feel like an abject failure.

"I wish I had never agreed to the surgery!"

We are committed, quite rightly, to advocate for our patients and treat them as we think they would choose if they were able. I just talked about strategies for helping the veterinary team deal with adverse outcomes. But the other major factor is the client. Not only do we want to help them understand, but we worry about being sued – or not paid – so we focus on educating them about their pet's disease, informing them of risks, giving detailed estimates, and getting signed consent forms. But we are not necessarily as good about helping them making decisions they can live with. If we wake at 2 a.m. and agonize over the way we treated Fluffy, how might Fluffy's owner agonize over sending their pet to her death?

Of course, Cathy Overall was devastated by Miss McGee's sudden deterioration, and that she would probably have to put the dog to sleep. She wasn't blaming us, she knew the risk she was taking, she was in no doubt about who had made the decision.

I wish I had never agreed to the surgery.

I felt terrible for her, anyway. I know what it is like to regret something. In Miss McGee's case

there was no taking it back. No rewinding and trying again. Cathy would have that with her forever.

Before Cathy signed the forms, I said, "You know that Miss McGee might die?"

Yes, she knew that. But she wanted to give Miss McGee the chance.

"I should never have done it," she said to me again, as she steeled herself to make the final decision for her companion.

Where did we go wrong? I wondered. I could not fault our professionalism, our science, or even the way we communicated the clinical information. Cathy might have been well informed when she gave her consent, but she was clearly not prepared for this outcome. How could we have equipped her better?

I understand why clients are upset when their pets don't make it. I never expect them to be *happy*. I have also seen how the anger stemming from their grief can be redirected, even when there is no real fault on the part of their veterinarian.

Perhaps the clinical discussion about risk factors was too abstract for Cathy. Perhaps she could not really imagine the way she would feel if the outcome was poor? Was there a way I could help future clients understand the true impact of the decision they were about to make?

Shortly afterwards, a retired couple brought in their Australian Cattle Dog, Betsy, for resection of a caudal abdominal sarcoma. After going through all the clinical aspects, I sat next to them and put my hand on the dog's neck. Betsy obliged by resting her head on my knee.

"This is a big decision for you and for Betsy," I said. "And once we start on treatment, we can't really go back. This is a fork in the road for her." I decided to spell out the scenarios very clearly. "If I do surgery, and it's successful, I know we're all going to be happy. Betsy will be able to enjoy her normal things, and she will send me a Christmas card."

They smiled. "We like that scenario."

"And I know if Betsy dies on the table, we will all be devastated …"

I paused. For the first time in the consultation, tears had appeared in their eyes.

Now you are beginning to "get" it, I thought.

"At least we will have tried," the female owner sniffed.

"There is another scenario we need to discuss," I said. "What if we do the surgery, and everything seems to have gone okay, but two days later Betsy has a complication and she is worse off than before? How are we going to feel then? And how are we going to decide when she has had enough?"

That took them aback. They could steel themselves to the idea of Betsy dying on the operating table, but the prospect of their pet suffering as a result of surgery, and having to make a decision to prolong treatment, or to euthanize her; that was something they hadn't even considered.

I don't like making clients cry. I don't set out to make it happen, but if that's what it takes to convince me that they have an inkling of how they will feel if things go wrong, then I feel I have done the right thing by them.

I used Cathy Overall's exact words. "I would hate you to feel you wished you had never agreed to the surgery."

The male owner said, "I don't know … I just … I don't know how I would feel."

"If you feel you might wish you had never done the surgery, this is the time, right here and now, to choose a different fork in the road." I continued. "If you think you could feel that way, it might be better that we don't go ahead."

The female owner said, "No. I would still feel that I had given her a chance."

I could see her husband was not yet sure.

"How about we give you a few minutes to chat," I said. "It is a very individual thing and there is no 'right' answer. I suspect everyone in this room – me, the resident, the student, the tech – might have a different response to that question. Most important is that you two understand one another, and that you feel you really are making the best decision for Betsy."

"Thank you," they said, and we left them and Betsy to contemplate a very unwelcome scenario.

When I came back 10 minutes later, they were determined to go ahead.

"We know we will be upset if anything happens," they said. "But we will be okay with it. We won't look back. Let's do it."

We did. And it went well. Four months later, Betsy sent me a Christmas card. She had excellent writing for an Australian Cattle Dog.

The question, "Do you think you might regret this decision if things go wrong," was powerful, and it definitely helped me to get things through to owners. But it still seemed a little abstract. I still thought I could do better.

I was fascinated to read Atul Gawande's book, *Being Mortal: Medicine and What Matters in the End*. The book covered many topics, with a focus on "how medicine can not only improve life but also the process of its ending."[3] Although I wasn't aiming to end my patients' lives, I did identify with some of the themes. At one point, Gawande addressed the concept of clearly identifying the patient's individual goals, and taking them into account when devising a treatment plan. What point is there in subjecting a patient to risk and pain for a very small chance of restoring athletic function, when what they really want is to watch their grandchildren playing in the yard? I thought this was especially relevant for my patients.

In Chapter 3, I introduced you to Ginger, the patient with extrahepatic biliary obstruction whose owner "just wanted surgery" – whatever the cost.

Rex's owner felt the same. Rex was a 16-year-old Dachshund with an invasive, but non-functional, adrenal tumor. The medicine resident came armed with a CT angiogram, expecting me to declare the mass non-resectable (Figure 14.1).

I examined the images carefully. I mentioned in Chapter 8 that I learned to visualize – and hence plan for – surgery when I was scrubbing, and as I gained more experience I became able to visualize a hypothetical surgery when someone

---

3 2014, Metropolitan Books.

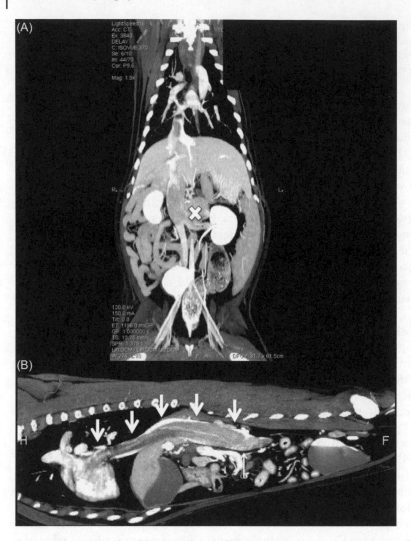

Figure 14.1 (A) Dorsal and (B) sagittal dual-phase computed tomography images of an invasive adrenal carcinoma (×) with a tumor thrombus extending into the right atrium of a dog (arrows). Courtesy of the Veterinary Medical Teaching Hospital, School of Veterinary Medicine, UC Davis.

asked me whether a case was operable or not. This was virtually a movie playing in my head. Sometimes, I would look at a CT and see only brutal dissection, bleeding, and unrepairable trauma. In this case, though, I could imagine dissecting around the adrenal tumor, opening the caudal vena cava, sliding the tumor thrombus out, and closing the incision again.

"Actually, I can't say that it's inoperable," I replied.

"Really?"

"Nope. I have removed tumors like this before."

"Wow. The owner will be happy."

"It's extremely risky," I said.

"They don't mind."

"Fifty percent chance of dying on the table."

"I told them that."

"Expensive."

"No problem."

"Are they ready for the other possible complications? Pancreatitis, regrowth, pulmonary thromboembolism?"

"I think so."

"How symptomatic is he?"

"Not at all, the ref vet picked this up when they did pre-op bloods for a dental."

It was a dilemma. I would love to do the surgery: it was challenging, and interesting, and always drew a crowd. I just didn't know whether it would help Rex for very long. "Is his owner comfortable with the idea of losing him, even when he is not showing any signs right now?"

"I'll go and talk to her again."

Fifteen minutes later, she was back. "When can you book him in?"

How long does she think dogs live? I wondered.

"Let's speak with her together," I suggested.

Before I entered the consulting room, the student briefed me in the corridor. "Monica is set on surgery. She told me she doesn't want anyone trying to talk her out of it. She says she knows the risks and she trusts us to do the best we can. She just wants to get things moving."

That seemed clear-cut, but I thought I should at least introduce myself. As I walked in, I reflected that my approach of running through "what if" scenarios might be fruitless with this client.

The student introduced me, "This is Dr. Hunt; one of the surgeons. Dr. Hunt, this is Monica."

Monica fixed me with a wide smile. "You're the one who is going to save my little boy!"

I smiled back. "I will certainly do whatever I can to help Rex." I knelt down on the floor and tapped my leg. "Hello, Rex. You're very handsome!"

Rex, who was sniffing happily around the corner of the room, trotted over, his undercarriage sweeping the floor. I patted him, then turned to the owner, "Sorry, I got carried away meeting Rex." I extended my hand. "How do you do?"

"Very well. When is Rex going to have his surgery?"

"We have him on the list for tomorrow. I know your doctor has talked to you about the procedure, and the risks ..."

Monica literally waved them away with her hand. "Yes, yes, we've been through all of that."

I thought on my feet. "I can see you are very dedicated to making sure Rex is given every chance ..."

"Yes, of course."

"So I just want to know whether you have considered all the possible outcomes from this surgery?"

"Well, I know he needs the surgery. He'll die if he doesn't have it." She looked me in the eye. "Won't he?"

I made a face somewhere between a frown and a grimace. "It's just ... he looks pretty happy and healthy at the moment."

"Yes, but how long is that going to last?"

"I don't think we can tell you that. It may be that his adrenal tumor grows slowly and doesn't cause a major problem. Or it may be that it gets big enough to make him feel bad quite soon. We are only seeing him at one point in time, so we don't know how long it has been there for and how quickly it will grow."

Rex did the rounds, greeting everyone in the room. He didn't seem to have the slightest idea he was suffering from a life-threatening disease.

I decided to try Atul Gawande's approach. "What are your goals for Rex?"

"I just want to the best for him."

"And how about your goals for *you*. What do you want Rex to be able to do with you?"

She considered this. "Just to be with me – for as long as possible."

Looking at Rex, it seemed that his quality of life was very good for a 16-year-old Dachshund.

Monica said, "I know he isn't going to live forever ..."

I spoke from the heart. "I'm not convinced we are going to improve Rex's quality of life much by taking him to surgery."

"But if I don't try ..."

I suspected we were getting to the truth now. Monica felt she would regret it if she didn't give Rex every chance. I tried another tack.

"You've told me that your goal is to have Rex with you for as long as possible. And you want to try and fix his problem, which means taking him to surgery. But we know we are not likely to cure him. The mass will come back eventually. So, from the risks of surgery that your doctor has discussed with you, are there any outcomes that would be intolerable?"

Monica looked at her little dog; curled up on the floor next to her foot. She scooped him up and he licked her chin. They might not have exchanged words, but they definitely engaged in some form of communication.

Eventually, she said, "He looks so well this evening. I don't think I could stand it if he died tomorrow, when I could have had him for a little longer." She nodded slowly. "That would be intolerable."

I didn't remind her that we were only giving him a 50% chance of surviving surgery. I didn't need to.

"I've decided," she said eventually. "I don't want to go ahead with surgery."

"Are you sure," I asked. "It will be even harder if you wait until he is showing signs, and then we try to do something."

"No, I'm perfectly comfortable. I wanted to make sure I had done everything possible for him, but I've realized I'm not prepared to lose him now, on the chance that he might live a few months longer."

We spoke a little more and I took my leave. I went back to the office and removed Rex's surgery request from the board.

"Really?" said one of our techs.

"Really. She decided she would regret it if he died on the table."

I had respected Monica's request. I hadn't tried to talk her out of surgery.

But some of our best surgeries are the ones we choose not to do. Despite the fact that I would have loved the surgical challenge, I am convinced that if Rex had died on the table, we would all have wished we'd never tried.

I now had a number of key questions for clients facing difficult decisions.

Will you wish you had never done this?
What do you want for your pet?
Are there any intolerable outcomes?

I was developing ways of encouraging them to think clearly about their goals, work out what eventualities they could and could not accept, and help them to make decisions everyone could live with.

Fearless Freddie presented a more complex challenge.

After speaking with the owner for over an hour, the oncology resident was downcast. "Mr. Badham just argues with everything I try to tell him. I really don't think he is listening to me."

Fearless Freddie (his nickname was Effy) had presented with coughing. Thoracic radiographs revealed a mass distorting one of his main bronchi. Effy was treated at another specialist center about a year previously for some sort of histiocytic tumor. Everyone suspected hilar lymph node metastasis, but we didn't know for sure.

"Did you ask him about 'intolerable outcomes'?"

"Yes. He says the only intolerable outcome is not knowing what the mass is, and wishing he had done more for Effy. He wants us to go in and take a look around."

"Us" meant "me," and "taking a look around" the heart base is not as easy as it sounds, and the dog probably had histiocytic sarcoma anyway. The coalition of a very tricky surgery, a likely poor outcome, and an intense owner who seemed refractory to discussion made me nervous.

"I don't feel good about this."

"Me neither. But he is adamant."

It was like a bad dream in which I could see the wreck coming but was unable to stop it.

"Oh, and one other thing. Mr. Badham told me he is a medical malpractice lawyer."

We decided to hold a multidisciplinary conference with Mr. Badham the following morning.

As I rode my bike home that night, I pondered the best way to approach the impending discussion. I had a bad feeling about it, but I didn't *know* that surgery was the wrong thing for Effy. If he had a primary lung tumor, it was resectable, and he recovered without complications, it might alleviate his signs and buy some reasonable time. But if it was a histiocytic sarcoma, how could we justify subjecting Effy to the risks and discomfort of surgery for very little reward? And it was presumably no accident that Mr. Badham alerted us to the nature of his profession, so we had the specter of being sued in the likely event things went sour. We could present Mr. Badham with a long list of risks, we could have him sign everything in triplicate, but was that really going to help if things didn't work out and he decided we were to blame?

I was also perplexed. Why did we seem more concerned about the impact of invasive treatments on Effy than his owner was?

Putting everything I knew about Effy and his owner together, I analyzed the situation and came up with a plan.

"Good morning!" I said brightly when introduced the next day. I was intrigued to meet Mr. Badham. Although many might consider internet "stalking" of clients to be unprofessional, I had been unable to resist googling him. I didn't find much about his professional life, but stumbled on the salacious tidbit that he had achieved fleeting notoriety three years earlier by water skiing naked on the Potomac River.

"I met Fearless Freddie yesterday," I said. I gestured to the gathered students, residents, and Faculty from Medical Oncology and Soft Tissue Surgery. "And we all discussed his case."

"You can call him Effy." Mr. Badham was shorter than I expected, with less hair, and quite rotund. The thought of him skiing naked down the Potomac River was …

I dragged myself back to the present for my opening gambit.

"It's great you came to us. You want state-of-the-art treatment for Effy and if it can be done anywhere in the world, it can be done here."

I don't know whether Mr. Badham was expecting to argue his point of view. Being a lawyer, I suspected he welcomed a vigorous debate, but I wasn't going there.

I proceeded to list the things we could offer Effy. Computed tomography, specialized anesthesia, intensive care, advanced surgery, blood transfusion, ventilator support.

"That's exactly why we are here," Mr. Badham agreed.

"And I know that finances are not a limiting factor."

"Absolutely not."

I looked Mr. Badham in the eye. "So we know we *can* do whatever Effy needs. What we have to work out is, *should* we?"

I was half expecting a quick "of course we should," but what I got was a moment's consideration. "Good point."

My window of opportunity had opened.

"I know you are aware of the risks involved in doing surgery. We might be able to help Effy, or we might cause a major problem."

"I know about the risks. But we have to know what this mass is."

It was like a waltz. Mr. Badham had followed my lead until now, so I followed him this time. "Yes, that would definitely help us work out the best strategy for Effy."

I had thought very carefully about this next step. "We can and will do whatever you want in order to help Effy. So, in my mind, the question really comes down to this: how much risk are you prepared to tolerate, in order to get some answers?"

In asking this question, I was hoping to shift focus from the logistics of the procedure, and from Effy himself, from us and whether we were able or willing to do the procedure, back to Mr. Badham. He was the one making the decisions, so he was also the one taking the risks.

It didn't absolve us of responsibility for doing the best job we could. It didn't change our liability should we make a mistake. It didn't reduce our commitment to Effy's well-being. But I hoped it would clarify to Mr. Badham that finding the best solution for his pet was not as simple as bringing Effy to a well-equipped hospital and opening his checkbook.

Mr. Badham opted for a CT scan. The CT showed a bronchial mass. It also showed several small nodules in the lung parenchyma. We couldn't tell Mr. Badham they were definitely neoplastic, so he remained adamant we take

Effy to surgery. The mass was so close to the hilus I had to remove the entire left lung field. Effy made a great recovery for 24 hours before he crashed. He became rapidly more dyspneic and required emergency intubation. Radiographs showed diffuse lung infiltrates. After three days on the ventilator another CT showed Effy's lungs to be uniformly abnormal. Histopathology confirmed disseminated histiocytic sarcoma and Mr. Badham decided to put Effy to sleep.

Do I wish I had never done the surgery? Absolutely – I didn't want to do it in the first place. But I would have hated to deprive Effy of even a small chance for recovery simply because I was scared to go ahead. I am sure I could have talked most clients out of surgery, but not this one.

After the initial awkwardness, though, Mr. Badham was unfailingly gracious. At the end, he thanked us effusively and registered the remainder of his fur family as patients of our hospital.

I don't know whether our conference with Mr. Badham made any difference to the way he dealt with us subsequently. Maybe he would have been at peace with his decision regardless of what happened. Maybe it simply made the veterinary side of Effy's team more comfortable about embarking on such a risky endeavor. Whatever the case, we navigated a difficult situation and came through with our professional integrity intact and the relationship with our client enhanced.

Maureen McGovern was right, "There's *got* to be a morning after." We are the ones who dictate whether it follows a good night's sleep.

15

One Leg Too Many

Patients Who Lost Limbs

The fire truck swung into the roundabout, siren blaring. Its lights were flashing and it really wasn't going all that fast, but it bowled Winston over, anyway.

Winston was just doing his rounds. Having more important things on his mind – like the scent from the café on the corner – and being used to sirens, he ignored the gaudy monstrosity until it was almost upon him. He had just enough time to jump sideways. Winston was not very athletic – thanks in part to his daily visit to the corner café – but that jump almost certainly saved his life. He didn't get very far, though, because one of the wheels had pinned his left hind foot. It then passed over his left front foot and – ignorant of the damage it had caused – the truck sped on to the fire, leaving Winston to wonder why he was unable to get to the other side of the road.

Winston arrived at our hospital with blood-soaked napkins around his injured legs. A Good Samaritan had abandoned her cappuccino and, with the aid of the barista, wrapped him in fine café linen and hoisted him into her car. We scanned his microchip as we evaluated the damage and Winston's owners were alerted.

"He's stable," we told them when they arrived, breathless and wild-eyed. "We've given him pain meds and oxygen, and put him on intravenous fluids."

"Bless you! Is he going to be alright?"

"There doesn't seem to be any internal damage. But he has injured two of his feet."

This was somewhat of an understatement. His left front foot was dangling by a strip of skin,

amputated just below the carpus. His back paw was still firmly attached to its limb, but had been ground to a pulpy mess.

"Will we have to put him down?" his owners asked.

We know dogs can lose two limbs and survive; the internet is peppered with images of all conceivable combinations. Given some natural athleticism, the right combination of walking aids, and dedication on the part of pet and owner, anything is possible. Winston was starting a little behind the line, though, as being a British Bulldog had gifted him with a number of orthopedic issues that made his remaining legs less than reliable.

We knew Winston's left fore was unrepairable, but was it necessary for him to lose his back foot as well?

We talked through options for the fore limb: amputate immediately, let the wound heal and fit a prosthetic, or send him away for a "bionic" leg.

"We can't afford that," the owners said. Amputation it would be then, once Winston was stable.

Now for the back foot.

The family held a conference. "No," they decided. "We won't amputate both legs." They would choose euthanasia in preference to having a two-legged dog. If there was any chance of saving Winston's back leg, could we please try?

We bandaged Winston's feet and let him stabilize overnight. We radiographed his chest, which was normal except for a cascade of hemivertebrae and a small hiatal hernia. We

Pitfalls in Veterinary Surgery, First Edition. Edited by Geraldine B. Hunt.
© 2017 John Wiley & Sons, Inc. Published 2017 by John Wiley & Sons, Inc.

radiographed his damaged back leg; no problem there except for his grade II luxating patella.

The following morning, we anesthetized him to inspect the damage. It was a simple matter to complete the transection of his left front paw and we opted to treat the stump as an open wound until we decided what to do with the hind leg.

Once Winston's back paw was cleaned up, the damage became more evident. The dorsal surface of his foot was split open, phalangeal bones splayed in all directions. His two middle toes were becoming necrotic, the nail of his second phalanx was pointing towards his carpus, and the fifth phalanx was completely absent. On a positive note, although his digital pads were rapidly dying off, his metatarsal pad was intact; flapping homelessly beneath the ruin of his metatarsophalangeal joints, admittedly, but intact.

I once struggled for weeks to save a cat's foot after a similar injury. She had not lost as much tissue as Winston, but the distal bones were pulverized. Although we achieved an excellent cosmetic result, the cat refused to use her foot and eventually developed draining sinuses. We ultimately diagnosed osteomyelitis and severe post-traumatic arthritis. She hopped around; miserable, lethargic, and losing weight; until we amputated her injured leg, upon which she raced straight to the backyard and began hunting birds again.

That case taught me to question the sense in undertaking heroics to save a limb a patient is unlikely to use again. So I like to make sure I, and the owners, understand our goals before we start the process.

For Winston, there was a particular imperative due to financial and clinical restraints. In the future, I hope we will have a more affordable range of distal-limb implants. But in this case, we were going to have to rely on his good old-fashioned natural healing process.

I once evaluated another cat, whose owners had found him hanging from a fence; his hind leg caught between two pickets. The owners suspected their neighbor, who'd expressed a hatred of cats in general, and Muggins in particular. Based on the difficulty we had even approaching Muggins – let alone handling him – I wasn't convinced; but that was neither here nor there. The foot was cold, but the cat was hypothermic and dehydrated so I admitted him for supportive treatment, and to see whether correcting his dehydration and hypothermia might improve circulation to his foot.

Sadly, the foot remained cold and insensate the next day, the nail beds a depressing pale purple color with no apparent refill. I even resorted to clipping one toenail short, but Muggins tolerated it without flinching and it yielded no blood whatsoever. The neurovascular bundle had been irreparably damaged and I amputated the leg.

Although the ruins of Winston's left hind foot had been cold upon arrival in the emergency room, it warmed up after being bandaged overnight. There was a continuous ooze of fresh blood from the damaged tissues and Doppler confirmed he had a pulse below the tarsus, while a neurologic exam prior to anesthesia revealed pain sensation.

Winston might not currently have anything resembling a functional weight-bearing surface, but his distal limb still had a neurovascular supply. Where there is life, there is hope.

I decided to remove all the visible bone fragments. I'm not an orthopedic surgeon, so I have less reverence for digits than my "hard tissue" colleagues. They have their uses, for sure – both orthopods and toes – but these digits had outlived their welcome.

Having debrided the obviously necrotic tissue, and removed the bone fragments, I was left with a relatively healthy-looking hindlimb with a slightly edematous flap of soft tissue at the end, the under-surface of which included the metatarsal pad and plantar interdigital skin (Figure 15.1A). We placed a wet-to-dry dressing and built a walking bar into a moldable splint. We changed the dressing daily for seven days, and when Winston began using his splinted hind leg, we performed a forequarter amputation of his front limb.

(A)

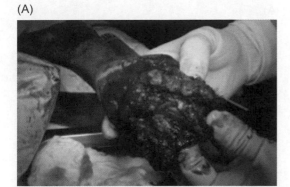

(B)

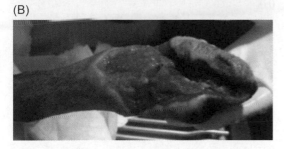

Figure 15.1 (A) Injury to the distal hind limb of a dog following motor vehicle trauma. All digits were destroyed, but the metatarsal pads remained viable. (B) The wound in (A) is healing well following open wound management. Granulation tissue contraction drew the foot pad under the stump to form a weight-bearing surface. This wound eventually closed spontaneously without surgical reconstruction.

The wound was granulating with minimal discharge, so we swapped to an absorbent polyurethane foam dressing, with silver sulfadiazine ointment to reduce bacterial contamination, and the owners brought him in every second day for a dressing change. In recognition of his hopefully temporary incapacity, the good citizens of the suburb in which he lived organized a daily roster to taxi him to the local café for his morning tea.

He sat in pride of place, just inside the front door, lapping his skinny puppaccino – now he had only three legs, he had to watch his figure – and displaying his war wounds.

"A *fire truck*? *Really?*"

Paparazzi followed his every move and he appeared regularly in the social pages.

Three weeks after being run over, Winston's foot was ready to be reconstructed (Figure 15.1B). At that stage, however, his owners ran out of money.

"Give us a couple of weeks to save up," they said. "We'll bring him back then."

We didn't see Winston for another month. When we did, he waddled into the waiting room. Winston had always waddled, but he now had a distinctly rolling hitch that brought to mind a heavily laden barge lumbering up the River Thames. His walking bar was gone. His splint was gone. He was using his "peg-leg" with gratifying efficacy. As the granulation tissue contracted dorsally, it had drawn the plantar skin and metatarsal pad neatly underneath the ends of the remaining bones and given him a weight-bearing surface. If you ignored the fact he had no toes, a star-shaped dorsal scar was the only lasting sign of the massive trauma that had been visited upon his foot.

"We were going to bring him in sooner," his owners apologized, "but the wound just kept getting smaller and smaller ..."

The surgery team quietly commiserated with one another. If only we had done the surgery before Winston healed himself!

The experience with Winston taught me not to be too hasty when condemning a foot. You need to have the right patient, and the right owners, and a perfused, innervated limb. And you can't be overly precious about maintaining anatomic correctness. But if it works, who cares?

I have removed and filleted many perfectly good second and fifth digits in order to close distal limb wounds, but the textbooks tell us that digits three and four are the major weight-bearing toes in dogs and cats and as such should only be removed when absolutely necessary. However, I knew how well Winston fared with *no* toes on his back foot, so I applied the same logic to my next oncologic patient.

Delilah's Grade 2 mast cell tumor had deployed itself directly between the two middle toes of her right hind foot. We discussed a marginal excision, followed by local irradiation, but we were all keen to try for a surgical cure.

"We'll almost certainly change her gait," I warned the owners. "And I wouldn't recommend that you enrol her for agility training. But I'm hoping she will still use the leg for the normal things any Boxer likes to do."

The owners decided that would be just fine as long as Delilah remained able to jump in and out of the car, as the thing she liked best in the world was to ride shotgun with her head out the window and drool on passing cyclists.

"No problems," I assured them.

I removed the mast cell tumor along with all the interdigital skin, and digits three and four provided the lateral margins. Then I reconstructed the cloven result with a phalangeal fusion, leaving her a bi-clawed stump complete with digital and metatarsal pads.

The result was so encouraging I did it again on Basil, the Doberman with a fibrosarcoma of the front foot, and Indigo, who had tangled with a lawnmower.

Billy Hughes, a West Highland White Terrier named after Australia's wartime prime minister, belonged to a human oncologic surgeon.

"It came up last week," his wife, Janice, told me.

"It" was a fibroma that had grown across the dorsum of the dog's metacarpus like an enormous plum (Figure 15.2A).

"My husband thought it would be too hard to remove, but then … we met someone at the dog park who told us you work miracles with feet!"

I loved the dog park. Admittedly, I only ever heard about the complimentary feedback that was exchanged on Sunday afternoons. I am sure there was the odd conversation, "*That Dr. Hunt, she mutilated Archie!*" but fortunately nobody ever shared it with me.

One lady brought her Weimaraner to me for spinal surgery after being recommended by a fellow dog walker.

"Her Cassie did *so* well!" the new client said. "The only problem was that for the rest of her life she could only walk down the stairs sideways."

I concluded this client had low expectations and for once felt under no pressure whatsoever.

(A)

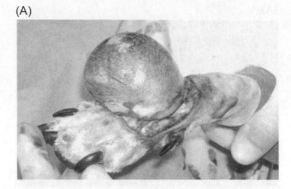

(B)

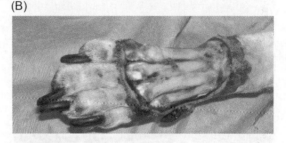

(C)

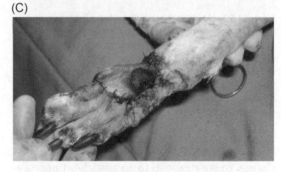

Figure 15.2 (A) Fibroma of the dorsal metacarpus in a dog. (B) The tumor was resected with a deep margin that included the common digital extensor tendons. (C) Skin flaps created by filleting the dewclaw and the fifth digit enabled closure of the excision site. The dog's owners grew fond of the repositioned fifth digital pad!

Billy Hughes' fibroma was a challenge. The mass was benign, but had grown rapidly and showed no sign of stopping. On further questioning, Janice admitted that it might have been there longer than a week, and that she'd had to twist her husband's arm before he would agree to surgery. The skin was very thin and discolored and I suspected it was one good lick away from ulcerating. It was time to remove it.

On the flip side, there was absolutely no available skin for closure, and no obvious deep margin. Did I really want to risk hastening the onset of a non-healing ulcer by creating an enormous wound? As an oncologic surgeon, Billy Hughes' Dad would know exactly what was possible and what wasn't.

Oh well, it was on record that I performed miracles with feet. How hard could it be?

I hatched a plan to resect the tumor and close the defect by filleting the lateral and medial digit. I drew a line diagram to show Janice how I would make the incisions and flap the skin over the top of the foot. It seemed like a good plan: it captivated the students and Janice liked it a lot. She told her husband, who wished he might be allowed to remove his patients' digits so glibly. I still had the issue of a deep margin, though.

"*The only way to be sure of a deep margin is to amputate the limb,*" I heard my inner oncologic surgeon tell everyone. The anatomist in me, however, was not so sure. I doubted the subcutaneous fascia was robust enough to provide a deep layer, although this was a benign tumor and therefore might be more forgiving. But there was a network of densely collagenous structures beneath the tumor that would provide an excellent deep margin if only I was brave enough to remove them.

"The digital extensor tendons!" my student assistant exclaimed when I told him.

I could imagine my professor saying, "*It will be interesting to see if that works.*"

Indeed it would.

"It will probably change the way Billy Hughes walks," I warned Janice.

"So would amputating his leg," she replied.

So I did remove the fibroma and the underlying extensor tendons (Figure 15.2B), and histopathology ultimately confirmed a clean margin. I then filleted the medial and lateral digits and reached that nerve-wracking point in so many reconstructive surgeries; where the hole is much larger than the available skin. The student went quiet as I stretched and shuffled the phalangeal skin flaps; in anyone's book, they looked pitiful.

"We can't suture them too tightly," I warned the operating room in general. Feeling less like a miracle worker and more like a butcher, I had resorted to the royal "we" to relieve my internal pressure. "We'll interrupt venous return and lymphatic drainage. The feet swell up really easily if we aren't careful."

No matter how much I rearranged and walked and stretched them, there was no way the two pieces of digital skin would close the surgical defect. There was only one thing for it.

"I'll have to leave the digital pad attached," I told the student. If the pad remained, I could close everything. I resected the distal ends of metacarpals two and five to remove an abrupt shelf, tapered the sharp edges with a rasp, and sutured the flaps together across the dorsal wound. The resultant hourglass effect made Billy Hughes' foot resemble a Edwardian socialite trussed up in a whalebone corset. And the disconcertingly waisted appendage was now adorned by an unsightly black lump (Figure 15.2C). Every time I looked at Billy Hughes' foot during the healing process, I had to remind myself that the dark spot was a digital pad and not an area of imminent necrosis.

"I can remove the pad later," I apologized to Janice. "Once everything else has healed and the skin has stretched a little."

Despite the fact that I had serious reservations during and after the surgery, it seemed I did work miracles on Billy Hughes' foot.

The first miracle was that he began using his newly shaped foot almost completely normally, despite the fact that he had no digital extensor tendons. I have to assume surgical scarring immobilized the tendon remnants enough to maintain the toes in extension and allow Billy Hughes to place his foot normally.

The second miracle was that the skin flaps survived and healed without complication.

The third miracle was that when Janice brought him back for suture removal the family had decided they would like to keep the digital pad where it was.

"It helps my husband explain how the flaps were created," she said. "And our friends find it quite hysterical!"

Having gotten away with resecting tendons in this dog, my options for oncologic surgery of the distal limb expanded significantly.

Fibrosarcoma of the metatarsus in an Irish Wolfhound?

"What structures are available for a deep margin?" I quizzed the resident of the day. I like to remind myself about the deep anatomy prior to resection, and identify the anatomic structures I might see on X-rays, ultrasound, or CT in order to plan the surgery properly.

I provided a clue. "There is a superficial and a deep layer."

The resident spoke softly, as if she were worried someone else might hear, "Digital flexor tendons?"

"Exactly!"

Unable to conjure a positive response, the resident went quiet.

I knew what she was thinking. We had gone to some effort recently to repair a partial Achilles tendon rupture in a Collie whose back toes were curling under his feet because the deep digital flexor was intact while the superficial digital flexor was not. Wouldn't we create exactly the same problem by resecting a perfectly good superficial digital flexor tendon in this patient?

"I am hoping the fact that Seamus' Achilles mechanism is intact means there is less tension on the remaining tendons," I rationalized.

"But what if it causes a gait abnormality anyway?" the student asked.

We basically had to choose between two conflicting goals: maintain normal function of the limb, or get rid of the cancer. The owners had already decided they wanted to try and save the limb if possible, although we warned them that if the histopath came back with a dirty margin, or the tumor recurred, amputation would be the next step.

"Would you rather have a dog with cancer, or a dog with a limp?" I asked them as they considered their options.

Not surprisingly, they chose the limp.

Now the resident mumbled something that sounded suspiciously like, "If he ever uses the leg again …"

Despite secretly wondering the same thing, I said, "Let's go for it!"

I then added insult to injury by having the resident perform the surgery with me watching from the sideline. At least I refrained from saying, "It will be interesting to see if this works."

Having encountered a bloodbath during a previous surgery in the same area, we placed a tourniquet of conforming elastic bandage, which allowed us to visualize the region better and carefully plan the resection and releasing incisions.

The surgery worked, and strategic filleting of the fifth digit provided a large enough flap to not only close the skin wound, but also reconstruct a defect in the metatarsal pad.

Seamus walked home on all fours the day after surgery and continued to use his leg in a normal enough fashion to make him a completely functional pet.

It was August, 1990, and the Gulf War had just begun. Our day was dominated by grainy news video of tracer bullets and exploding bombs. I was trying to focus on an exploratory laparotomy and having a hard time of it. I finished the surgery and left the operating room to an immediate beep from my pager. Could I come to the treatment room and look at a dog's leg? It was urgent.

The medical team were clustered around an examination table occupied by a brindle-colored Greyhound. The Greyhound's left hind foot was bandaged.

"He came in this afternoon," the registrar told me. "The owners took him interstate for a race. He split the webbing between his toes and was stitched up at the track two days ago. But he hasn't used the leg since and now they're back home they wanted us to check it out."

Not using the leg at all didn't sound good. Infection, most likely, resulting from poor hygiene at the track.

"Show Dr. Hunt what we found," instructed the registrar, and the student peeled the bandage away.

Rather than being swollen and inflamed, the foot was pale. The skin looked macerated, and smelled awful. This was more than infection; it was rampant necrosis. Necrotizing fasciitis had not yet been reported in the dog, but we were aware of a rare condition where the soft tissues started to die off, and this was high on our list of differentials.

The registrar continued grimly. "Show Dr. Hunt what else we found."

The student removed the rest of the bandage. I gasped, and not just because of the foul smell.

Wrapped tightly around the limb, just above the hock, was a makeshift tourniquet.

"Oh, no!"

Somehow, for some inconceivable reason, the vet who stitched the split webbing had placed a tourniquet and then omitted to take it off.

Even as I struggled with how on earth we might manage this situation, the medical registrar began to unwind the tourniquet. In retrospect, we should have done it slowly, placed an IV catheter and started fluids in the event that toxic substances were flushed back into the dog, even considered doing something to prevent reperfusion injury. But we were so unnerved by the circumstances that all we could think of was to remove the tourniquet as quickly as possible.

Amazingly, within a few minutes after the tourniquet was removed, color returned to the footpads and blood began dripping from the suture holes in the digital web. The dog did not seem concerned by what was happening, apart from swinging around and trying to lick his delightfully – for a dog – fragrant foot. Later that night he would chew off his toes.

"I think we'd better phone the interstate vet," I said.

"Already on it," replied the registrar. Her resident returned very soon afterwards, "He's booking a flight over here."

Needless to say, the Greyhound's owners were unimpressed a tourniquet had been left in place under the bandage. Even less impressed that, despite resumption of blood flow, the entire distal limb continued to necrose. Finally, as a three-legged Greyhound is a poor racing prospect, they opted to euthanize the dog but then agreed to surrender him in the hope that we might find him a home.

The interstate vet paid the costs of treatment and exhibited his concern about the situation by flying in the following morning. I was in surgery and never met him, but did hear more of the story.

It seemed he had placed the tourniquet, stitched the webbing, and then been called to the telephone, leaving the nurse in charge of placing a bandage and waking the dog up. It was simple, really; he was busy and did not have a safety net. He didn't blame the nurse; he took responsibility and paid the entire cost of evaluation and amputation.

From that day onwards, I began to identify my patients in some way when I placed a tourniquet, an anal purse string suture, pharyngeal swabs, or ideally anything else we did not want to accompany the patient to the recovery room (Figure 15.3).

Although the Greyhound's owners could have made a good case, I never heard of any subsequent legal action, which suggested the dog had not covered himself in glory on the track. People in our town had recently discovered that Greyhounds made excellent pets so the local adoption network did its thing and this particular Greyhound appeared to miss neither his hind leg nor his testicles as he hopped off to a new home. A number of Greyhound cadavers had been found in local landfill with the

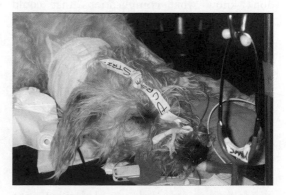

Figure 15.3 Safety label on a dog's head indicating that a purse string suture has been placed in the anus and alerting staff to remove it once the procedure is finished.

identifying tattoos on their ears cut out, so it is possible this medical misfortune saved him from an early death and a shallow grave.

There are many ways we can cause our patients to lose a limb: Ehmer sling too tight; the owners didn't bring the dog in quickly enough for bandage change after elbow luxation.

We caused compartment syndrome by suturing the skin too tight after removing a crural mast cell tumor. I talked about sciatic nerve damage following perineal hernia repair in Chapter 5. In that case, it was reversible, but if it hadn't been … tripod time.

Jade, the Beagle, presented with polyuria and polydipsia. Her referring vet was thorough and in addition to blood tests – which showed hypercalcemia – they performed a rectal examination. Bingo! Jade had a pea-sized anal sac adenocarcinoma, and golf ball-sized sublumbar (medial iliac) lymph nodes.

"Can you get it down to microscopic disease?" the oncologists asked.

I looked back sceptically. The CT showed massive lymphadenomegaly all the way along the hypogastric chain. I could feel the most caudal one projecting between the tail and the anus.

"Please!" Jade's owners begged. They had come to me because I was *"willing to have a go."*

"You know she might bleed to death on the table. I might ligate major blood vessels and I don't know what complications that could cause. Or I might damage the nerves to the bladder or anus and make her incontinent."

"We know. We know."

"Are you sure you're ready to lose her?"

"No. But we know she isn't going to last long if we do nothing." This was certainly true.

"You won't regret this decision if things go wrong?"

"No. And if she is worse after surgery we will let her go. At least we will have tried."

As there was no "standard" incision for this decidedly non-standard case, I decided on a combined abdomino-perineal approach. We placed Jade on her back in a gently frog-legged position with the hind legs drawn forward to tilt her perineum upwards. Her tail hung off the very back of the table. I first made a laparotomy incision extending back to the pubis and explored the pelvic inlet. My resident and I removed the medial iliac lymph nodes with moderate difficulty using blunt dissection with the LigaSure™.[1] Although they were nestled between the great vessels, it was possible to peel them away, giving me hope the intrapelvic nodes might be equally forgiving. Leaving the resident in the abdomen, from where he could palpate and manipulate structures at the pelvic inlet, I made a U-shaped incision dorsal to the anus. Dorsal recumbency was not the ideal position for this approach, but being able to access the pelvic canal in this way was very helpful.

I had also considered a pubic osteotomy, but as the nodes were largely dorsal I preferred not to try to shift the urethra, colon, and neurovascular structures out of the way in order to see what I was doing.

"Maybe nodes will just fall out."

My students laughed dutifully, not believing me for a moment. But they hadn't been there in other cases, where I had been able to grasp the node – or another type of tumor – with my fingers or a pair of Allis forceps and, after gentle probing of the surrounding tissue, literally pluck it from the fatty abyss (Figure 15.4).

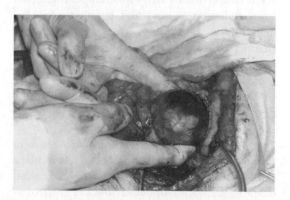

Figure 15.4 "Plucking" a leiomyoma from a dog's pelvic canal using gentle digital dissection.

---

1 LigaSure™, Covidien, Boulder, CO, USA

Either these lymph nodes would shell out, or they would be soldered onto the structures around them. After a few minutes dissection, I realized that they were not the "pluckable" type.

Jade's owners had been absolutely clear on their goals of surgery.

"I might get to a point where it is 'do or die,'" I said. "If I go ahead, we risk major complications."

"That's alright. Do whatever you possibly can."

The pelvic nodes were sessile and very firm. When I tried to grasp them with a forcep they fragmented. They had broad attachments to the sacrum that made it impossible to manipulate them enough to see the adjacent structures. I could push my finger cranially, and the resident pushed his caudally, but the lymph nodes remained immobile. If they had just been attached to the sacrum I would have been less concerned, but they were almost certainly encasing the terminal branches of the aorta. Fortunately, dogs have excellent collateral circulation, which means we can get away with ligating much larger blood vessels than human surgeons, whose patients often have peripheral arterial disease in addition to their sparser vascular distribution. But ligating the terminal aorta would be pushing our luck way too far.

I was charged with removing the lymph nodes at all costs to the dog and the client. What did we have to lose? Having established there was seemingly no intolerable outcome for Jade's parents, who urged me to be as heroic as possible, I now had to decide whether I had any intolerable outcomes.

What about the personal cost to me?

We hear about compassion fatigue in veterinary science and other caring professions. The more dogs we put to sleep, the easier it gets. The more pain and suffering we see, the less it affects us. The less we care. The topic of euthanasia came up in a social setting once, and new acquaintance said to me, "Oh, well it wouldn't worry you, vets do it all the time!" I realized there was a huge disconnect between what the public would *like* vets to be – caring, dedicated people who devote their life to the profession because they love animals – and the impression some people seem to have – callous scientists interested mainly in research and making money. I have euthanized many patients. I have conducted research; in many cases using animal subjects. Did it make me care less about the cat I was putting to sleep, or the sheep in whom I was implanting an experimental pacemaker? Maybe early on, but not later. Not now. I came to realize that every life I took, and every complication I created, exacted a toll on me. Maybe that is also true for others? It may be a toll we can afford, or it may be one that bankrupts us. But there is a toll, and we do well to remember that.

So when Jade's owners asked me to remove her lymph nodes *at all costs*, I recognized that their conviction applied to them and to Jade, but not to me. I was the only one who could decide whether I was prepared to undertake something that might take a toll. It made me think, *What costs are acceptable?*

I could have said no to the whole exercise. I have refused to do surgery in other cases, and other surgeons had told the owners that surgery for Jade was hopeless, which is why they came to me. If Jade had been suffering the effects of advanced cancer, or she was constipated due to the mass effect; if she had not been hypercalcemic; I might also have refused. But her clinical signs were referable to her hypercalcemia, and I knew that reducing her tumor mass – if possible – could buy her some quality time. So I agreed to try, but now needed to work out where I would draw my personal line in the sand.

I decided I could accept losing Jade perioperatively as a result of bleeding.

I could also accept leaving fragments of lymph node in situ even though I had been charged with removing everything (which I never thought feasible, anyway).

I could accept a wound dehiscence or even wound infection. I would follow good surgical principles and apply all my experience to the task, and hopefully minimize the risks within my control.

I could even accept postoperative necrosis of the pelvic organs if I was unable to identify critical blood vessels within the resection zone and Jade's collateral flow was insufficient for adequate tissue perfusion. Her condition would deteriorate and we would have to put her to sleep, but I had already established that Jade's owners had a low tolerance for added pain and suffering – despite their aggressive approach – and they would make the decision if it seemed Jade was not recovering well.

What I was *not* prepared to tolerate, I decided, was random hacking and slashing. Perforating or transecting the colon or the urethra, for instance. Removing things that I *knew* would create major disability, as opposed to doing a resection that *might* lead to complications.

Having established that, it seemed the best first step was to identify the urethra and rectum and take steps to ensure they were not damaged; structurally, at least.

I placed a urinary catheter (relatively easy as the dog was in dorsal recumbency). Then I fed a stomach tube through the anus and into the colon to identify the bowel. At each stage of the dissection, I checked that the urethra and colon were safe from the scissors, LigaSure™, or surgical clamps. The masses separated fairly easily from the pelvic viscera, but remained firmly attached to the dorsal pelvic cavity. I tried levering one off with a periosteal elevator and was rewarded with a rush of arterial blood that left me in no doubt as to its relationship to the median sacral artery.

Does the tail necrose if you cut the median sacral? I wondered.

After pushing and pulling, poking, prodding, and levering, I realized the only way I was going to be able to shift these fibrocartilaginous neoplastic concretions was to run the LigaSure™ between them and the sacrum and burn the heck out of whatever connected the two. Which is what I did. I burned and cut, and burned and cut, until the jaws of the instrument were caked in sticky char, the surgical field resembled a barbeque hotplate, and the room was filled with a faint smoke haze. Eventually, I drew the chain of

lymph nodes from the perineal wound, leaving a large tunnel that allowed me look through the perineum and see my resident's fingers in the caudal abdomen.

Through it all, I protected the rectum and urethra as best I could in a shroud of moist gauze reinforced with malleable retractors.

My spirits fell a little when the resident retracted the caudal abdominal viscera (my hands were contaminated from my perineal exertions so I kept them well away from the laparotomy) to reveal the LigaSured stump of a large vein.

"What is that?" I wondered out loud. "And more importantly, what artery goes along with it?"

The students found somewhere else to look; if I didn't know what it was, they certainly didn't want me to start quizzing *them*.

We knew it wasn't the caudal mesenteric. Being an unpaired vessel, and providing a critical blood supply to the colorectal junction, the caudal mesenteric artery had been one of the structures we had guarded with our lives.

"Iliac?" ventured the resident?

"*Internal* iliac," I agreed, hoping it wasn't. The internal iliacs supplied most of the pelvic viscera. I inspected the vessel more closely. It seemed that it was just the vein; the artery was still embedded in fatty tissue. I tried to remember how many internal iliacs a dog had and polled the audience. The general feeling was that they must have two. The median sacral was the only unpaired vessel going to the back end.

I asked the resident to unwrap the terminal colon and rectum and we inspected it for any sign of congestion. It didn't look overly happy, having been retracted for an hour or more, but it had capillary refill and contracted when pinched.

"Internal iliac vein," I decided, and we moved on. We lavaged the abdomen and the pelvic canal until I was standing in a serosanguinous soup peppered with flakes of charcoal. Having created an impressive hernial ring dorsally, I sutured the anal sphincter to the coccygeus muscles on either side, and the resident closed the abdomen routinely. Then we crossed our fingers.

Jade's owners and the oncologists made me feel like a hero when I told them the news. Her blood calcium level was noticeably lower after surgery and continued to drop in the days following surgery. Blood-stained diarrhea oozed from her anus for a day – making me paranoid about the integrity of her rectal mucosa – but quickly resolved. Jade seemed comfortable and began eating within a few hours of surgery. Her wounds failed to dehisce, her tail did not die, and she was able to urinate normally. All in all, she made a miraculous recovery.

Except for the fact she could no longer use her left hind leg. It had a great pulse, but that's where the good news stopped. Somewhere in all that mess of dissecting and cauterizing, I transected her sciatic nerve: or more likely, the nerve roots.

I had gone through so many different risks in my own mind and with her owners, but this one had completely escaped me.

Jade's owners didn't seem to care. The dog couldn't even feel her leg, so she wasn't especially worried, either. She started chemotherapy and visited the Physical Rehabilitation service before each of her oncology appointments. They trialled slings and orthotics and carts, but eventually settled on suspending the useless limb in a sock hung from a tape around her belly. As far as Jade's owners were concerned, her left hind leg was a perfectly good trade for the extra year of life surgery brought her.

And the personal toll was one I happily paid, in order to give Jade that chance.

16

Reconstruction Rescue

When the Hole Just Keeps Getting Bigger and Bigger

I wish I had invented the phalangeal fillet surgery,

It is so anatomically nifty and, in addition to providing me with many hours of fun, has yielded superb clinical results. I also wish I had thought of the cosmetic nasal reconstruction technique described by Gallegos, Schmeidt, and McAnulty.[1] I've only been able to try it once, but it made me feel like the best vet in the world!

Reconstructive surgery for oncology captivates me because it brings some of the most rewarding features of soft tissue surgery together in one patient: anatomy, the challenge of the resection, creativity in repairing the defect, and satisfaction when the wound has healed. Moving skin around so it seems nothing has ever happened can also stroke your ego nicely as your colleagues study the wound for clues as to how you worked your magic.

For all those truly brilliant reconstructive outcomes, however, there is an equal number of less rewarding ones. And although you might think that the surgeries early in your career are the ones most likely to fail, when I look back through the retrospectoscope, I realize that – at least for me – that wasn't the case.

Admittedly, the complexity of the cases I tackled increased in proportion to my level of experience, and a case that I might have found intimidating early on barely raised my heart rate a few years later. But I never lost that flush of satisfaction when I successfully created even the simplest skin flap.

My first reconstructive triumph was a middle-aged Standard Poodle called Neige. An apricot-sized fibrosarcoma had appeared on the lateral aspect of her left knee. I decided to recruit loose skin from the medial aspect of the stifle and create a flap based roughly over her patella.

"Abracadabra!" I cried, as I seized the edges of the skin flap and pulled it firmly over the defect. My student assistant gasped, but sadly not at my conjuring powers.

Oops!

I already knew – based on Laurie, my first-ever surgical case – that soft tissue surgery is far more forgiving than orthopedics. But it doesn't forgive poor preparation, and once you start making releasing incisions, and pulling in skin to close defects, you learn that the extra skin has to come from *somewhere.* In pulling Neige's skin flap tight, I also dragged her flank fold into the surgical site and, although only sparse, it was hirsuite nonetheless. I never imagined I would need to clip and prep the skin *that* far away from the incision.

There wasn't much we could do at that stage other than call for an emergency prep of the area that had been exposed.

"Spray plenty on," I instructed the surgical nurse. We were using iodine and I knew it was inactivated by organic material, but hair in your surgical field is far less disturbing when you have stained it brown.

---

1 Gallegos J, Schmiedt CW, McAnulty JF. Cosmetic rostral nasal reconstruction after nasal planum resection: technique and results in two dogs. *Veterinary Surgery* 2007; 36: 669–674.

Pitfalls in Veterinary Surgery, First Edition. Edited by Geraldine B. Hunt.

That done, I continued pulling the flap in the direction I intended it to stretch. The skin around the excision site had retracted so far that it was disappearing under the drapes, and the new skin flap was shrinking before my eyes. It looked like it would be large enough when I made the incision, but seemed sadly inadequate when relocated to the front of Neige's knee. It didn't seem to know whether it was an advancement flap, a rotation flap, or possibly even a transposition flap. In the end, it had elements of all three, including a lateral extension to the incision that proved redundant, and which I then had to suture back together again.

"Let's take the drapes off and see how it all looks," I said to the student. As we did, it became evident the resistance I felt when trying to move the skin flap was not due to inherent tension in the skin itself, but because it was being immobilized by the way I had positioned the towel clamps. Once we removed them, we liberated a generous piece of stretchy skin that would have made closure a piece of cake.

I had now learned two lessons: *be careful when positioning towel clamps* and *clip further than you think you'll need*.

"We can check how much tension there is on the wound," I informed the student, grasping Neige's back foot and moving her leg back and forth. The hip and stifle flexed without any restriction. I began to extend the hip, but the skin stretched drum-tight across the front of the stifle. I had positioned Neige in lateral recumbency for the surgery, and her leg ended up slightly flexed. I was able to close the defect without tension in that position, but in doing so had restricted Neige's range of movement. Now, each step she took would drag the skin wound apart.

I added point 3: *make sure you can move the leg through a complete range of motion before you close.*

You can't feasibly do that in some wounds because of the way you have to position the patient, so I later modified that rule to *try to position the limb for the "worst case" scenario.* I would far rather have a dog-eared or crumpled skin flap than one resembling cured parchment.

That aside, I still felt a great sense of achievement with Neige's completely closed wound.

"My first skin flap," I said proudly as I paraded her past the primary care clinician who sent her my way. He was very generous in his comments, but I suspect that was because he found lying more tolerable than watching a grown woman cry.

Neige was, of course, a white Poodle. The flood of emergency iodine – coupled with meandering blood stains – made her look almost quilted. When her incisions finally healed, they formed discolored furrows and the hair on the areas I had actually shaved grew back a dirty gray color – as well as pointing in odd directions. In short, through every stage of the surgery and recovery, you could see exactly where I had been.

My first skin flap quickly became my first dehiscence. Not because the blood supply was inadequate; the base was almost as wide as the flap was long. Probably not because of infection, although I deserved it after my poor surgical prep. No, my downfall was tension, and this would continue to be my biggest challenge for years to come, until an even more fiendish adversary declared itself.

The smell of decay preceded Asterix as he was led into my examination room. Serosanguinous fluid escaped a makeshift "nappy" and dripped between his back legs.

"What a beautiful boy!" exclaimed the student, who had clearly blitzed her doctoring class.

I greeted the owners with a forced smile, wondering how they had managed a three-hour drive without resorting to gas masks. Asterix took an immediate shine to me and bounded over, rubbing his unseemly rear end around my leg and dripping on my foot.

Endeavoring to display similar compassion to my student, I clutched at the best compliment a surgeon might make in this situation.

"He breathes really well for a French Bulldog!"

Perhaps I was projecting forward and imagining the multiple instances of sedation and anesthesia in Asterix's future. I clearly wasn't convincing enough because the owner said, "It smells bad, I know. Is that normal?"

The owners reported that Asterix had staked his right inguinal area about 10 days ago when out playing in the local reserve. It tore open a ragged, 8-cm degloving wound of the flank fold. His local vet cleaned out the obvious fragments of wood and sutured the skin over a Penrose drain. Regardless of the quick attention, the wound started to discharge and broke open, then continued to weep profusely after resuturing, at which stage Asterix was referred to us.

"It's hard to keep bandages around the inguinal region clean," my student explained without prompting. "And if they get soiled with urine, or fluid from the wound, the bacteria can grow in there and smell pretty bad."

Quick thinking and diplomatic; this student was potted gold! But I was fairly sure the smell coming from Asterix could mean only one thing. It had a character quite different to the fruity rot of *Pseudomonas*.

"Is it alright if we take him to the treatment room and get him cleaned up?" I asked. "Then we can evaluate things and talk to you about how we can help."

Like flies descending upon a carcass, the smell brought a number of heads popping around the treatment room door. Most of them disappeared just as quickly, curiosity dampened by the fact that the smell was, indeed, coming from a patient, and that it wouldn't be dissipating any time soon.

"Why do we think the wound might have dehisced?" I asked the student in charge of Asterix, and those other robust souls who remained to watch the unveiling.

"Because it stinks."

I laughed, "No. I mean, what caused it to dehisce?"

"Infection."

"Poor blood supply."

"Tension."

"Foreign body?"

"Potentially all of the above," I agreed. "It might not have been possible to avoid this. In fact, I would probably have treated it the same as the local vet, if Asterix had been brought here. But I would have warned the owner there was a fairly high risk of dehiscence, regardless."

The resident unwrapped the bandage and my audience retreated as the putrescent odor intensified.

"Hmmnnn ..." The resident peered between Asterix's back legs, then inspected one flank, followed by the other. "This is odd."

Rather than one large defect, as we were expecting, we saw a network of sutures extending from the left flank, across the caudal abdomen, and down the medial aspect of the right hind leg. The caudal sutures were springing apart and a large piece of weirdly fenestrated gray skin clung to the inside of the right thigh.

Necrosis; you have to love the smell of cadaverine in the morning.

She said, "It looks almost ..."

"Meshed," I finished. In fact, it looked remarkably like a skin graft.

Try as we might, we couldn't reconcile the wound the owner described with the one we were seeing now. The situation was complicated by the fact we had not received any written records from the referring veterinarian.

I am embarassed to admit I often left the other members of the surgical team alone with unpleasant tasks like cleaning a rotting wound until it was in a fit state for me to evaluate. Today I felt more benevolent.

"Why don't you see if you can get the vet on the phone?" I suggested to the resident.

She made a quick exit, presumably before I had a change of heart.

"Can I stay?" the gold-plated student requested. While the other students recoiled, she was leaning in, seemingly anosmic.

"Of course."

Regardless of how the defects were created, it was clear we had a large cavity in the inguinal fat pad and a necrotic flap of skin, both of which would have to be debrided and treated as open wounds before we could even think about reconstructing them.

We flushed away the discharge and dried the area off. Once the sodden bandage and the worst of the mucopurulent discharge were removed, the general miasma of decay dissipated and Asterix began to smell more like a patient and less like a pathology specimen.

It took three days to get the whole story; that didn't disadvantage Asterix, because we couldn't do much in that time beyond open wound management. A wound culture spawned a similar spectrum of organisms to what we might have grown from the dumpster outside our lunch room, but they were all sensitive to amoxicillin/clavulanic acid.

As best we could work out, the vet who did the wound repairs forgot to write a surgical report before he left for vacation in the Solomon Islands. There was an undue amount of tension when he tried to suture the original wound. He decided a rotation flap would help close the defect, and took the flap from the medial aspect of the right leg. Unfortunately, both the original wound and the flap donor site then dehisced. At that stage, he decided to resuture the original wound and perform a skin "graft" to close the flap donor site. He created the skin graft by recruiting a transposition flap based on the right skin fold, then rotated it – still attached to the trunk – and made many small releasing incisions in order to stretch it across the open medial wound. When this still didn't close the wound, he added a free graft. This explained the necrotic pieces of skin clinging to the inner thigh (Figure 16.1). He then ran a Penrose drain under the skin from the inguinal area to the tarsus.

"He was very excited," his colleague told me. "He said he'd never done a mesh graft before!"

"Unfortunately it necrosed."

"Oh, man! Why do you think that happened?"

Where to begin? I thought. I framed my answer carefully. The vets' response would depend entirely on whether they really wanted to know what to do differently next time, or simply needed reassurance that they were not to blame for the complication. I decided to give them the benefit of the doubt, and answered as honestly as I could.

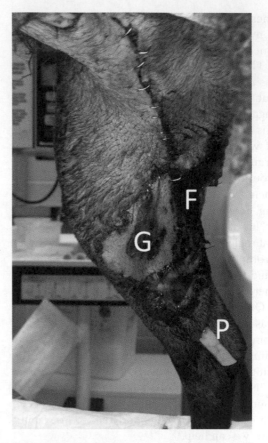

Figure 16.1 Wound dehiscence with necrosis of a free skin graft (G) and a meshed pedicle flap (F) on the caudomedial aspect of a dog's leg. Free grafts must be carefully immobilized to encourage adhesion to the underlying tissue. This graft probably became necrotic as a result of local movement, complicated by presence of a Penrose drain (P) under the graft. The pedicle flap was probably devitalized as a result of tension and disruption of the subdermal plexus when it was meshed.

"It's a high tension area so movement is always going to be an issue. Skin grafts don't have a blood supply of their own and so they are completely dependent on contact with an underlying wound bed. If there is any movement, or if the wound bed isn't healthy, they are likely to fail. The Penrose drain probably caused some elevation of the graft. It is very hard to immobilize skin grafts in the upper limb at the best of

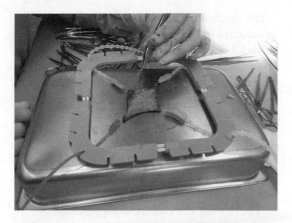

Figure 16.2 Dissecting the subcutaneous tissue during preparation of a free skin graft.

times, and this graft was still attached to the leg, so each time the dog moved its leg, it would have pulled on the graft."

"But he left it attached to its pedicle, so it would still have some blood supply …"

"Yes, a *pedicle flap* is reliant on the subdermal plexus blood supply for survival. In removing the subcutaneous tissue, and meshing the skin, you destroy the subdermal plexus and turn a flap into a graft. A graft has to absorb plasma from the wound bed, so you have to remove all the subcutaneous tissue (Figure 16.2). You have to decide which you are creating: either a free mesh graft, or a pedicle flap. In this case, you got the worst of both worlds: movement, and a disrupted blood supply."

"So you *would* have treated the wound differently, if you'd seen Asterix right at the beginning?" the student asked me in rounds.

I had thought a lot about that since I learned the details of the case, and discussed it at length with the resident, so I let her answer.

"I would have tried to be clear about our goals at each stage," she said. "Our first goal was to decontaminate the wound and close it if it seemed healthy enough. But if the skin edges were too badly damaged, we might have left the wound open for a couple of days before trying to close it."

"And how about the rotation flap?"

"I think it was premature. If there was too much tension on the wound while it was still contaminated, then we would have left it open. We wouldn't have done a skin flap until we were pretty sure it would heal properly."

"What about when it dehisced, would you have used a skin flap then?"

"No. At that stage the wound is showing you it isn't healing properly. So doing a skin flap would only increase your risk of making things worse."

"How long should you wait?"

"Wait until the wound is either starting to granulate, or at least until you know there is no ongoing necrosis and it doesn't look overtly infected."

"And the skin graft?"

I repeated the things I told Asterix's veterinarian.

Asterix had an open wound for a long time, but once the necrotic tissue was debrided it granulated rapidly, and contracted surprisingly well, and we placed a loose continuous suture in the skin to allow us to start bringing the skin edges together by applying a little extra tension each day; sneaking the edges closer while the granulation tissue did its thing underneath. And although we set Asterix's owners up for another reconstructive effort once everything looked healthy – they were understandably nervous about this, as were we – we never had to do it.

My resident sat on the floor of the surgery office, staring at Bilbo. Bilbo stared back. A Dogue de something-or-other, he had a Mastiff's impressively large head and a generally crumpled appearance. Despite those generous folds of skin, which should have ensured that any surgical defect could be closed without tension, he had a large, granulating wound caudal to his left elbow.

I was not surprised when they told me his mast cell tumor excision site had broken down. I didn't trust mast cell tumors, even when they had been removed with 3-cm margins. Another colleague claimed there was no proven association between mast cell tumor excision and poor wound healing, but I felt I knew better.

As it turned out, when I finally did a retrospective study of our surgical cases to prove the association between poor wound healing and local heparin or histamine – or some other evil effluvium of these ubiquitous neoplasms – I found nothing of significance.

Whether or not it was cause and effect, there was certainly an association in Bilbo's case. Excise mast cell tumor – end up with gaping hole on lateral thorax. We had been treating this dehiscence as an open wound for three weeks now. It had granulated nicely and even begun to contract, but by virtue of repeated wound cultures we had seen its microbial colonists morph from innocent bystanders that fell over at the sight of a beta-lactam to seriously evil villains with rapidly evolving drug resistance. Now, we were faced with the unpalatable necessity of placing a cephalic catheter and starting ticarcillin.

We had hit a speed bump, however, in that Bilbo's owners were rapidly running out of cash.

"The bandage changes alone are costing a fortune," my resident lamented. "And I haven't even tried to calculate the cost of Timentin in a 63-kg dog."

Bilbo began panting and raised his head; huge jowls flopping back to reveal fluorescent mucous membranes.

"Whatchou laughing at, mister?"

His bright red mucous membranes were not a sign of sepsis; in fact they were anything but. Despite being "infected" with one of the scariest bacteria in the hospital, Bilbo was one of its happiest patients; afebrile, eating like a horse – he probably ate *more* than many ponies – wagging and drooling happily when taken for walks, and – more importantly as far as his owners was concerned – peeing and pooping up a storm. Less so, his student, sentenced to the hard labor of barrier nursing and the meticulous cleaning commensurate with Bilbo's methicillin-resistant status.

"They want to know when he can go home."

I considered this for a moment. "Is there any reason *not* to send him home?"

The resident, student, and tech stared at me as though I had gone mad.

"He's happy. He wants to go home." I didn't know the right answer to the question, but in talking through it perhaps we would work it out.

"But the infection ..."

I frowned. "What evidence do we have that the wound's infected?"

"It's been infected from the beginning."

"We treated the initial infection. But is it infected now?"

"That's what the culture is suggesting."

"True. But Bilbo doesn't seem to know that. He isn't febrile, the local tissues aren't inflamed, he isn't in pain, and he's eating normally."

The student spoke as though I had just decoded the Rosetta Stone. "Do you mean we don't need to worry about the infection?"

I wasn't going to say that. We had gone to the trouble of culturing the wound; wouldn't it be culpable to ignore the results?

I deflected the question. "What are our goals in treating the infection?" I asked the gathering in general.

A couple of mouths opened, and then closed.

One student ventured, "To make sure the wound heals properly ..."

"It looks like it's healing to me."

"To make him feel better ..."

Bilbo grinned at us.

"Are we treating the patient?" I asked, "or the culture report?"

"Yes, but ..."

It is that "*yes, but*" that makes it so very hard for us to exercise responsible antimicrobial stewardship. Yes, but – *what if we don't treat the infection and Bilbo becomes septic?* Yes, but – *what if the wound doesn't heal and the owners are angry with us?* Yes, but – *what if I don't treat it and stay awake at night wondering whether I should?*

None of which changed the fact that when I looked at Bilbo, the *only* compelling reason I could come up with for giving him ticarcillin was because we had cultured a certain type of bacteria from his wound.

I continued my train of thought. "It seems we have a local problem, rather than a systemic one – does everyone agree?"

They did.

"So, why not look at ways of treating it locally?"

There are any number of products with activity against bacteria that you can use locally on wounds: silver, methylene blue, gentian violet, chlorhexidine. In Bilbo's case, we had a decent "*out*" in that the owners were not in a position to pay for daily treatment with parenteral ticarcillin. But they could probably afford a tub of silver sulfadiazine. This wasn't a choice between whether to treat or not to treat; this was an exercise in working out which compromises could be both reasonable and ethical.

"So, let me ask the question again. Is there any reason not to send him home?"

"He's still having daily bandage changes."

Bilbo's bandage changes were quite the exercise; everyone wearing white gowns and gloves, the techs laying disinfectant-soaked mats at each doorway, and all the resultant debris being consigned to an infectious waste bin. Not to mention the rolls and rolls of absorbent padding and Elastoplast.

"Couldn't the owners do bandage changes at home?"

"Could they do the barrier nursing?" added the student who by now had received far more training in that area than she could ever have wished.

"They don't need barrier nursing at home. We are doing that for our protection – not for his."

"I doubt they could apply a decent bandage. We're finding it hard enough to get them to stay on as it is."

I wasn't trying to suggest that I was cleverer than everyone else; I was honestly thinking through this dilemma out loud. "Why are we doing all these bandage changes?"

I suspected I already knew the answer to this one. We were doing bandage changes because *that's what you do when you manage something as an open wound.*

This wound had progressed past the effusive phase, so it no longer needed a highly absorbent bandage. Indeed, much of the expense with our current bandage changes came from applying a non-adherent contact layer to avoid it sticking when the absorbent middle layer dried the wound out too much. The gist of the subsequent conversation clarified that we were bandaging this wound for three reasons:

1) to protect it from the patient
2) to protect it from the environment
3) because it looked ugly.

And we weren't even doing those three things very well, because the bandage often slipped, requiring costly replacement.

"I'm not suggesting we shouldn't treat infections," I clarified to the group, "or that there is anything wrong with state-of-the-art bandaging materials. What I am suggesting is that you think carefully about *why* you are choosing a certain treatment. Make sure you clearly understand your goals for treatment, and ensure the treatment you choose is really necessary to fulfil those goals.

"Can't we work with the owners to design a bandage they can change at home that would do all the things we want?" I asked.

"They could apply silver sulfadiazine regularly," the resident mused. "And use an old T-shirt, or maybe some stockinette to cover the area. Something cheap that they can secure in place, but also remove more easily than Elastoplast. Something that won't require a hospital visit if it slips."

"Shall I phone the owners and see what they think?" asked the student.

Bilbo went home that afternoon.

We saw him a week later to confirm that his wound continued to look healthy. We warned the owners that should Bilbo appear unwell he would have to come back in for antibiotic treatment.

It took two more weeks of contraction before we were brave enough to discontinue the Silvazine and the T-shirt. We decided not to culture the wound again.

No reconstructive surgery, no ticarcillin, no professional bandage changes, no hospitalization with barrier nursing; it seemed that I was doing myself out of a job. Would we have done things differently if Bilbo's owners had all the money in the world? Probably.

Would it have been better for Bilbo? I'm not sure.

What I am sure about is that the escalation of bacterial resistance during my career forced me to think more and more creatively and flexibly about how I approached wound infections. It seemed that any patient with unresolved soft tissue disease would eventually grow methicillin-resistant organisms. Open wounds, ulcerated tumors, otitis externa, skin fold pyoderma; you just needed to give them a long enough course of antibiotics. Then bring the patient into hospital, keep them there for elaborate and lengthy treatments, and you can contaminate your other patients as well.

It seems counterintuitive to combat an increasingly complex disease with progressively simpler strategies, but sometimes we are left with little alternative.

When I graduated from veterinary school, the mainstays of antibiotic treatment were penicillin, chloramphenicol, streptomycin, and sulphonamides if you were in large animal practice. Clavulanic acid came on the scene and Amoxil gave way to Amoxy-Clav – or Clavamox, Synulox, or Clavulox, depending on where you were practicing. Chloramphenicol fell out of favor because it was bacteriostatic and could cause aplastic anemia. Sulfonamides were regulated to the halls of history and gentamicin was superseded by the fluoroquinolones. Even infections that remained susceptible to penicillin began to be treated with clindamycin and metronidazole.

So I thought it ironic – as we cast around for an alternative to ticarcillin and vancomycin – when we discovered that Bilbo's twenty-first century superbug was also susceptible to a drug discovered in 1947.[2]

"These bacteria haven't seen chloramphenicol for decades," our biosecurity officer explained. "So we can start using it again." He paused. "Carefully. And with regular blood counts."

I would love to tell you that I discovered some surefire ways to avoid wound dehiscence, but I would be lying. And I would love to reassure you that once you are experienced enough, your wounds won't dehisce any more, but that would be another fib.

Are there things we can do to reduce the risks of dehiscence? Almost surely. Will we always need a plan for when wounds dehisce? Absolutely.

I was listening to a lecture by my friend and colleague – the "wound guru" Bryden Stanley – some years ago and she impressed upon me the importance of being gentle with skin edges. If it was good enough for William Halstead, it was good enough for us. It made me think about the way I handled the tissues during reconstruction. I realized that in trying to undermine, relocate, and extend skin, I handled it a *lot*. I picked it up with forceps, skewered it repeatedly with towel clamps, and stretched it as far as I possibly could (Figure 16.3). I let the subcutaneous tissue dry out, cauterized the heck out of everything, and generally traumatized all I touched.

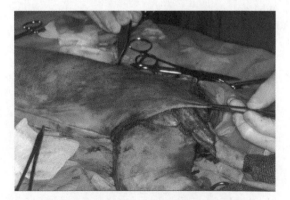

Figure 16.3 A demonstration of how *not* to hold skin while moving flaps around during a reconstructive procedure. Try to grasp the subcutaneous tissue rather than the skin edges to avoid small strips of necrosis.

2 Maviglia R, Nestorini R, Pennisi M. Role of old antibiotics in multidrug resistant bacterial infections. *Current Drug Targets* 2009; 10: 895–905.

It was no wonder – when I looked back through my surgical excisions from the past half-decade – that I discovered almost half of the patients with skin flaps went on to have some degree of wound dehiscence; worrisome enough to mention in a discharge statement. And in looking at additional risk factors, there was a strong association between the length of the surgery and the incidence of dehiscence. It made sense. The longer you fiddle with the tissues, the more damage you do. Prompted by Dr. Stanley to actually look, I acknowledged that 2–3 mm at the edge of my skin flaps often turned black and peeled away. The edges might not have died back enough to cause full-thickness skin dehiscence, but they were clearly unhappy. Dryness, manhandling due to repeated grasping, and stretching all seemed likely culprits. I began strategically using skin hooks, and I tried to grasp the subcutaneous fibrous tissue rather than the skin edge itself when manipulating the flap. And I developed a very low tolerance for skin stretching. Rather than tensioning the very end of the flap, which was probably clinging on for dear life, anyway, I would start at the base of flap, where the tissues were closer to their collateral circulation and might have a better chance of surviving.

Think about pulling on a wetsuit. Simply stepping into it and pulling it up by the shoulders doesn't work very well – for most of us at least. It stays baggy around the knees, tugs annoyingly at the crotch, and is unbearably tight around your neck. Better to start with the legs and tension it evenly all the way up, making sure it fits snugly at each level, so that at the end you can comfortably pull it over your shoulders and zip it up without asphyxiating yourself.

For those of you who don't dive or surf, think about pulling on your surgical gloves. The fingers are the base of our imaginary skin flap and the wrist is the distal extremity. We don't just grasp the open end of the glove and pull it over our fingers; there is too much inherent resistance and we end up with a very tight fit around the heel of our hand while our digits are awry, competing for the flopping fingers and rarely finding the right ones. This is exactly what happens if you suture the distal end of your skin flap first, without spreading tension from the base.

Ideally, when donning our surgical glove, we try to seat our fingers comfortably first, then spread the tension through the rest of the glove towards our wrist. Likewise, when securing a skin flap in position, I begin suturing at the point of greatest tension close to the base, and ease the flap toward the defect, taking up a little more strain with each bite, stretching the flap more evenly and protecting the vulnerable distal end. If you've planned your flap properly, once the base is immobilized you can lay the flap in the defect and have it stay there without retracting more than a few millimeters. If you can do that, you know that once you complete the suturing, the distal end of the flap will be under minimal tension. This works best if you can use your subcutaneous layer to take all the tension, and use your cutaneous sutures simply to get a leak-proof seal between the skin edges.

Of course, it stands to reason that if you place *any* part of the flap under a lot of tension – including the base – you risk interrupting its blood supply at that point, in which case the distal end could be as relaxed as a Copacabana beach bum and it would still necrose.

Try these techniques; they will make for a more comfortable snorkeling experience. They may even reduce the amount of time you spend treating wound dehiscences and actually allow you to get down to the beach!

17

"Why Is Sam Straining?"

Iatrogenic Strictures and Stray Oddities

"I'll wager this case is right up your alley!" Bernie led a nervous-looking Kelpie cross into the treatment room. The dog walked stiffly; head low and lip folds tasseled with saliva. "He ate a chicken wing yesterday."

This was in the weeks after I finished my PhD.

Right up your alley, referred to my newly gained experience with thoracic surgery, and *he ate a chicken wing yesterday* suggested Bernie was betting on an esophageal foreign body. I didn't know whether to be excited or terrified.

"I'm going to take a chest X-ray." Bernie ushered the dog into the X-ray room and closed the door. I resumed trying to find a retained testicle in an inguinal fat pad the size of a bowling ball.

Neither of us was successful. Max's chest X-ray was normal and I learned that I wasn't going to find Boomer's errant testicle by shredding the fat pad; I needed to be more strategic.

"I have to go. Caitlyn's got netball practice." Bernie handed the Kelpie and a urine collection cup to our sole nurse. "Can you take him out for a pee then put him in a cage? I told the owners we would do some tests and call them later."

Karen and Max disappeared into the backyard. Entrusting my own patient to the Ap Alert – our only monitoring device at the time – I turned my attentions to his inguinal ring. By the time nurse and Kelpie reappeared, both testes were in the trash and I was closing.

The urine cup was empty. Karen apologized, "He wouldn't do anything."

I finished closing, switched off the anesthetic machine and carried Boomer to his cage. "I'll see if I can palpate a bladder."

Max's bladder was much easier to find than Boomer's retained testicle. It was huge.

"Did he even try to urinate?"

"No, he just stood there groaning."

With two more desexings to do before a full afternoon of consulting, I decided to cut to the chase. Karen held the wriggling Max while I passed a urinary catheter. It didn't go very far. Back to the X-ray room and we had our answer; a log-jam of radio-opaque urethral calculi just caudal to the os.

"Pearls of the penis!" Karen declared.

Slightly less excited, I performed a needle cystocentesis, drained over a liter of blood-stained urine, and Max sank to the floor like a deflated helium balloon. The guinea pig castration and the Rottweiler spay would have to wait while I went pearl-diving.

"Max has stones in his urethra," I told his owner over the telephone. "He needs surgery to remove them."

"His urethra? I thought he had something stuck in his chest?"

Clearly it has migrated. I kept the thought to myself.

"No, the chest X-rays were clear, but I passed a catheter up his urethra and found the blockage."

The owner sounded impressed. "He let you pass a catheter up his urethra!?"

"Yes. I can't say he liked it much, but he let us do it."

Max's owner gave permission for surgery and I went ahead with a cystotomy and urethrotomy. Having never done this surgery before, I phoned

Pitfalls in Veterinary Surgery, First Edition. Edited by Geraldine B. Hunt.
© 2017 John Wiley & Sons, Inc. Published 2017 by John Wiley & Sons, Inc.

Bernie for advice and he suggested leaving the urethrotomy wound open to granulate in order to reduce the chance of a stricture. Max recovered smoothly and without complication except for three things:

1) Mrs. "Max" failed to tell Mr. "Max" about the quote for surgery, so he had an acute attack "sticker shock" when he came to pick the dog up the next day. So nauseating was the experience, in fact, that he threw up in the flower bed outside reception.
2) Having recovered somewhat, Mr. "Max" lodged a complaint that I had passed a urinary catheter without using any local anesthetic because catheterization was so painful. (I considered this an over-reaction until many years later when I experienced the agony for myself.)
3) Because Max was intact, his temporary urethrostomy led to skin maceration and an ugly scrotal dermatitis that may well have been more painful than anything else he experienced.

Max taught me many lessons; none-the-least being that we should *always* do a thorough physical examination before jumping to conclusions. The next most important was that – commonplace and simple as it might seem – urethral catheterization is a delicate procedure to be carried out carefully, and with due concern for your patient's comfort. Not only can you destroy a trusting relationship, but the urethral mucosa can and will tear if you are not gentle with it.

When we decide to pass a urethral catheter we usually have a good reason and probably can't just shrug and walk away if it doesn't go into the bladder, so we have no choice but to persevere, and progressive disappointment leads us to become frustrated, distressed, and rough – usually in that order. Urethral trauma is probably more common in our patients than we recognize and – after seeing a string of cases with urethral complications following deobstruction by veterinarians – I developed a very high index of suspicion for rupture or stricture in patients presenting with repeated or ongoing difficulty

urinating. The risk of obstruction at the level of the os penis resulting from inflammation, trauma, or stricture leads many vets to recommend permanent urethrostomy if they have to retrieve stones from that location. Although some vets recommend simply leaving the urethrotomy site open to avoid stricture, I feel a meticulous closure should achieve the same end. On the other hand, because of the potential for male dogs to form cysteine and oxalate calculi repeatedly, you might also decide to perform a permanent urethrostomy and reduce the risk of future obstruction. My experience with Max made it clear that castration – by means of scrotal ablation – and a scrotal urethrostomy provide a superior result to pre-scrotal urethrostomy if you do choose not to close the urethra. Having been forced once to do a perineal urethrostomy (PU) in a male Rottweiler with osteosarcoma of the corpus cavernosum, I can attest the scrotal approach is definitely preferable to the perineal if you can possibly manage it!

The urethra is vulnerable where it passes around the ischial arch and turns cranially into the pelvic cavity. Urinary catheters do not slide naturally around this corner, so either use a very flexible catheter or place a finger at the ischial arch (just below the anus) and apply gentle pressure through the skin to guide the tip dorsally and then cranially to avoid having the catheter follow its instincts into the perineal subcutis.

Partial-thickness urethral trauma can also lead to a valve-like effect, where things pass antegrade but not retrograde *or* – more problematic – retrograde but not antegrade (i.e., you are able to catheterize the bladder but the dog still can't urinate). Consequently, I do lots of positive contrast urethrograms (Figure 17.1).

Benson the St. Bernard was so huge we had to commandeer a stable in the horse barn. Following three days in another hospital for treatment of a gastrointestinal upset, he had not peed on his own for over a month. We could express his bladder with ease (he would allow this as long as you kept well clear of his food bowl, in which case he would roar and rush at

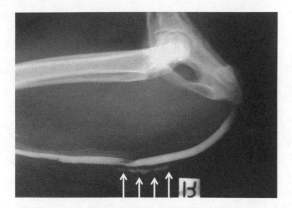

Figure 17.1 Contrast urethrogram showing urine leakage (arrows) following urethral rupture as a result of repeated attempts at catheterizing a male dog.

you with jowls flapping and teeth like walrus tusks). We could pass a catheter without any problems – using a muzzle. But squat and strain and creep and trickle as he did, Benson could not even begin to empty his bladder, which had now inflated to the size of a football. Ultrasound and contrast urethrography probably should have yielded an answer, but these were early days and he was a very large dog with a very short fuse, so we couldn't confirm any diagnosis apart from a suspicion that he suffered urinary retention in hospital and his detrusor muscle had packed it in. A variety of vesicular "upper" and "downer" drugs did little to help[1] and, as any form of handling became progressively more stressful – not to mention dangerous – for doctor and patient, we decided to place a cysto-stomy tube.

I took the opportunity to explore Benson's urinary tract in the process. The apex of the bladder looked as suspected; distended and dis-colored, wall compliance similar to cured leather. Being such a huge dog, my initial inci-sion was woefully inadequate, and although I had incised well caudal to the prepuce, I was still

at least 5 cm away from the pubis. I couldn't even feel back to Benson's prostate, so I extended the incision through the centimeters of fat that gradually divorce the penis from the caudal abdominal wall in aging male dogs. The caudal-most portion of a laparotomy incision can be confusing, as the extra-abdominal fat is similar in texture and appearance to the paracystic and periprostatic fat pads near each inguinal canal. It can be hard to know whether you are in the abdomen or not, especially if your incision starts caudally. For this reason, I like to enter the abdomen near the umbilicus and extend the incision cranially and caudally once I have confirmed I am through the peritoneum. In Benson's case, his bladder was distended and just seemed dysfunctional until I retracted the abdominal wall cranial to the pubis, palpated the urethra just cranial to his prostate, and sepa-rated the fat along the midline to get a better view. The vesiculo-urethral junction was pinched tight, and I had to completely deflate the bladder before I could manipulate the tissues enough to see that Benson's bladder had torsed 180 degrees.

I don't know whether the torsion was chronic or acute; I don't know whether it resulted from repeated manual expressions, or whether the bladder just went floppy as the obstruction became more chronic, predisposing it to displacement; I also don't know whether the torsion was permanent or only temporary. There was no necrosis, no areas of dubious perfusion, and Benson was pissed-off but not painful when we palpated his abdomen, which was very different to the two cases reported over 10 years later.[2] I am certain, however, had I not explored the very caudal-most portion of

---

1 The drugs we used, their dosages, and mechanisms are not relevant to this story. This happened a long time ago and there are many excellent contemporary references to help you. My aim is to share my experiences with decision-making and surgical pitfalls – not internal medicine or pharmacology.

2 Pozzi A, Smeak DD, Aper R. Colonic seromuscular augmentation cystoplasty following subtotal cystectomy for treatment of bladder necrosis caused by bladder torsion in a dog. *Journal of the American Veterinary Medical Association* 2006; 229: 235–239.

Thieman KM, Pozzi A. Torsion of the urinary bladder after pelvic trauma and surgical fixation. *Veterinary and Comparative Orthopaedics and Traumatology* 2010; 23: 259–261.

the abdomen, and made sure I actually visualized the region – which required some commitment because of the voluminous fat pads – I could easily have placed the cystostomy tube without recognizing the bladder malposition, which would have ensured Benson never urinated normally again. I would like to tell you that Benson's detrusor muscle recovered as completely as Mungus' did in Chapter 11 but I can't, because a week after we placed the cystostomy tube he pulled it out, and soon afterwards became lost to follow-up.

Samson was endearing in the wriggly, ballistic way eight-week-old kittens have perfected. He was normal in every respect except for spending his formative years in his litter tray. He had some sort of urethral obstruction that precluded passing a urinary catheter and had reached the stage where he was only surviving by virtue of daily cystocentesis. But Samson had no owners, and his foster parents did not have very deep pockets. He had come to me to be evaluated for a PU. I had never been asked to do one in such a young cat before, but it seemed it was probably Samson's last hope. That is, until Dr. Julie Meadows walked in with a very important question. "Shall I book a table for this evening?"

Dinner at the local restaurant had become a regular tradition, especially on Thursday nights when everything on the wine list was half price.

"Not sure; I might be operating on this little critter." Samson was amusing himself by chasing his tail around the leg of a chair. Then he stopped mid-loop and attacked his rear end. "He can't pee," I explained.

"Preputial stenosis?"

"What?"

Julie repeated, "Does he have preputial stenosis?"

I had never heard the term before. "He has some sort of stenosis. His vets can't pass a urinary catheter. He's come in for a PU."

"May I?" Julie swept the kitten up and peered beneath his tail. "Yes, looks like it to me. The littermates cause trauma by suckling one another, and the inflammation leads to scarring and stenosis." She turned the cat's butt towards me. "See?"

I was amazed; I had never heard of this condition before, and possibly still wouldn't know about it had it not been for Samson and Dr. Meadows. A literature search turns up scant references to the condition in cats,[3] and Dr. Google is equally unhelpful. It seems this condition is one you must learn about by word of mouth.

We anesthetized Samson in the afternoon and confirmed he had a pinpoint preputial orifice at best. Being an institute of higher learning, we found a way to pay for a radiographic contrast study that showed a large collection of urine within the preputial cavity. We could have done a full urethrogram using minimally invasive techniques but time and money were running out, so we decided to fix the obvious problem first. I managed to ease a flexible surgical probe through the stenotic preputial orifice, slide it in a centimeter or so, and elevate it to act as a firm landmark palpable through the skin. In principle, this is identical to the open technique described for anal sac ablation. Taking care to identify each layer as I went, I incised the skin from the preputial orifice radially, using the probe as a guide, until I could see subcutaneous tissue. Then I used fine scissors to divide the fat and underlying preputial mucosa. An encouraging fountain of urine sprayed from the defect onto my fenestrated drape. The tip of a very normal looking kitten penis popped into view. Now I could see what I was doing, I was confident to enlarge the incision until I felt the orifice was large enough to heal without stricturing again.

"Would you like to do the honors?" I passed the student a Tomcat catheter. The catheter slid into the penis and on to the bladder with minimal resistance, yielding a second font of gold.

"Woohoo!" I couldn't help myself. Three hours ago, Samson was looking at euthanasia. One tiny incision and now he could pee again!

---

3 Hun-Young Yoon, Soon-wuk Jeong. Surgical correction of a congenital or acquired phimosis in two cats. *Journal of Veterinary Clinics* 2013; 30(2): 123–126.

I used very fine (5-0) absorbable sutures to appose the incised edge of the preputial mucosa to the corresponding skin incision. The key factor in preventing and correcting strictures is careful apposition of epithelial surfaces. Leave gaping holes to granulate, and you will find granulation tissue does what it is designed to do; contract. If that happens circumferentially around a wound, the wound gets smaller. So will an orifice like a urethra, tracheostomy, or external ear canal. It is one of the reasons I am so keen on placing my patients in dorsal recumbency for a PU; it allows me a great view of the dorsal-most anastomosis site, and the area where it is most critical to do a good job.

When I was finished, Samson's prepuce resembled a wide keyhole from which the reprieved tip of his penis jutted joyously (Figure 17.2).

Rather too joyously, I thought, hoping it would behave more demurely once the surgical inflammation settled. But none of us were really worried about cosmetics right now, for when we removed the urinary catheter and squeezed Samson's bladder a prodigious stream of urine arced right across the treatment table. Everyone in the room cheered except the work experience student, who fluoresced with embarrassment at the wet patch Samson had so generously hosed onto the front of his scrub pants.

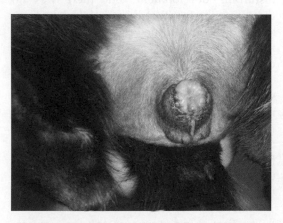

Figure 17.2 Jubilant penis and edematous mucosa following surgical preputioplasty in a kitten with preputial stenosis.

I consoled him by pointing out that it meant Samson would probably do just fine.

PU is one of those surgeries you can learn to either love or hate. My early boss, Bernie, managed with no magnification, no assistant, and minimal lighting. His results seemed remarkably good, although I know of at least one occasion when the procedure gave *him* a migraine. I can't say I approached them with the same confidence, at least not initially. Perhaps because I found the procedure so daunting, and thus took extra care, I didn't cause a major complication until long after I became a specialist.

Wally was a big ginger boy brought low by frequent episodes of urinary tract disease. His bladder created so much sand we had to send in a figurative dredger each time he started to strain. After repeated bouts of obstruction and a variably successful trial of medical management – Wally's housemate was being served far more palatable meals which Wally stole two times out of three – we made the decision to perform a PU.

By now, I found PUs fairly non-threatening and rewarding, although we (the profession in general) were beginning to recognize a considerable risk of long-term complications. But if it could keep your patient out of hospital and avoid those disheartening battles to keep a urinary catheter in place, it seemed worthwhile for all parties.

Wally was duly prepped and placed in the perineal stand and I commenced the teardrop incision around his prepuce.

Having done this surgery often enough to acquire a healthy dose of hubris, I made a half-hearted attempt to catheterize the tip of Wally's heavily silted penis then decided I could do it easily enough through a urethrotomy. I incised the skin, reflected the retractor penis muscle, exposed the corpus spongiosum, and incised in the direction of the urethra. The tissues bled profusely and digital pressure did little to help. I cut deeper with a No. 11 scalpel blade and the ooze of venous blood became a stream, clearly escaping from a cavernous vessel. It appeared I had missed the urethra altogether.

"Hold this," I instructed the student, clamping a wad of surgical sponge over the defect and pressing her finger into it. I returned to the dangling prepuce and exteriorized the tip of the penis. I still could not pass a urinary catheter, but I could at least start incising the urethra from here. I inserted one blade of my sharp iris scissors into the urethral opening and began splitting it open by incising through penis, subcutis, and skin; all in one go. Once the caudal aspect of the prepuce was completely divided, I pushed the scissors up towards the original incision, still being diligently compressed by my student. Having identified the urethra at that site – by now the bleeding had settled to a dull roar – I demonstrated the next stage of the procedure.

"Now I will place a mattress suture across the penis to control bleeding, and amputate the end of it." I matched words with actions, and discarded the tip of the penis and prepuce into the trash, leaving us with a stump of penis and transected urethra.

"I will continue splitting the urethra dorsally." I slid the iris scissors further into the visible opening in the stump of the penis. A rivulet of dark blood ran down the blades and dripped off my hand and onto the floor.

"Ah, that must have been the corpus cavernosum again," I squeaked. Hubris was rapidly giving way to humility, with its accompanying prickle of perspiration. I inspected the stump of the penis again. I could see nothing resembling the transected urethra, and I couldn't work out why the corpus cavernosum was on the caudal aspect. I was tempted to blame Wally for having abnormal anatomy, but realized it was more likely that the penis had twisted 180 degrees when I was placing the mattress suture. I twisted it back and forth, had the student place pressure on it for another couple of minutes, and eventually found the urethra again by random probing with a urinary catheter. This time, I was able to feed the catheter cranially, to the great relief of both myself and Wally's bladder. The surgery tech predicted what was to happen next and politely fiddled around my feet as she spread an incontinence pad onto the floor. I let the catheter drip urine and used it as a guide to incise the urethra up towards the pelvic canal.

Then I palpated the left crus of the penis, where it attached to the ischiatic tuberosity, slipped my scissors across, and cut it. A minute or so of digital pressure controlled the bleeding and I did the same on the other side. Now I had the urethra separated from its boney attachments – just as the textbooks describe – and hanging in space. I continued the periurethral dissection far enough to identify the bulbo-urethral glands, covered by a thin layer of urethralis muscle. I could see the flayed end of the urethra, so it was a simple matter of incising it until I reached the widened pelvic portion.

"Oh!" The student grabbed for the catheter as it slipped out. She just missed and it landed on the pee pad.

"Don't worry," I said. "The urethra is much wider now so we shouldn't have any trouble seeing it now. Here we go." I found the opening and slid the scissors forward carefully, but admittedly with a small flourish.

The entire penis came away in my hand; connected to the cat by a translucent slip of subcutaneous tissue.

"Oops." My instinctive outburst caused all heads in the room to swivel.

I didn't particularly want to confess to this disturbing development, but there was no disguising the fact that I was holding the transected distal end of the urethra, and the proximal end had just disappeared into the pelvic cavity.

I thought everything was progressing just fine so this came as a complete surprise, but surgical mishaps are often like that. Having mulled over it thoroughly, I eventually concluded that the urethra must have twisted again as the catheter fell out. Instead of making a linear incision in the urethra, I made a spiral one that eventually transected the whole thing.

What do I do now?

The first thing I did was ask for a sweatband, as the precipitation from my brow intensified.

After much probing, I was able to pass a urinary catheter into the pelvic stump of the urethra and through to the bladder. I grasped the friable tissue surrounding the urethra and pulled it caudally to achieve a fragile urethropexy. But I was not able to confidently suture urethral mucosa to skin, and although I left a urinary catheter in poor Wally for two weeks, the stoma strictured and I eventually had to salvage him by means of a prepubic urethrostomy. I submitted his penis and distal urethra for histopathology, which showed a florid urethritis. The urethritis might have contributed to my surgical difficulties, but I think my main mistake was not to have a urine catheter in position through the whole procedure.

In my next PU, I also added the security measure of placing a suture on the caudal aspect of the penis so I could make sure it did not twist. I liked the strategy of incising the urethra from the tip of the penis (*work from the known to the unknown*), and from then on I always left the prepuce attached until I had identified the pelvic urethra. Nowdays, I do the procedure in dorsal recumbency (just as I do for perineal hernia; see Chapter 10), which improves visualization of the tricky dorsal mucocutaneous anastomosis and allows access to the abdomen and bladder if needed.

I would almost certainly have needed to flip Wally over and open his bladder had I not been able to catheterize the pelvic stump of the urethra once it retracted, but had I positioned Wally in dorsal recumbency, I might also have had some more options, like squeezing his bladder to see where urine flowed from the urethral stump, or even opening the abdomen and passing a guide wire or catheter antegradely to help identify his urethra. With intraoperative flurosocopy, it can be done in a minimally invasive way.

Although prepubic urethrostomy yielded an acceptable outcome in Wally, I always thought I might have been able to do better, and he flashed back into my mind many years later when I read Bernarde and Viguier's excellent paper on

transpelvic urethrostomy in cats.[4] They described an intuitive approach to accessing the pelvic urethra that capitalizes on the anatomic features of the region and allows a major modification to be made without compromising function.

If only I had thought of it!

When Alicja began straining, her owners searched the internet for an explanation and shortly thereafter rushed her to the vet to unblock her bladder.

"How long has this been going on?" he asked as he palpated Alicja's abdomen.

"About a month."

"Her bladder feels fine, but she is quite constipated."

After reassuring the Wojciks that Alicja did not have a life-threatening emergency, their vet prescribed a laxative and suggested they feed her a soft, moist diet for the next few days to get things moving.

It didn't work; Alicja passed feces regularly, but they were ribbon-like and did not come out easily. After another couple of months, her parents were ready for referral.

"Megacolon." The student tapped the computer screen – I like digital radiographs; no more greasy fingerprints smeared across the area of primary interest, or crayon marks giving away the roentgenographic punch line. It certainly did look like megacolon; painfully distended with the speckled, radio-opaque gravel of chronic obstruction. Alicja was very young for megacolon, but it was not unheard of.

Her owners were distraught. They searched megacolon and returned; armed with over 100 pages from the Google library. Diet had failed. Acupuncture hadn't worked either, nor chiropractic. Alicja was becoming progressively more and more unwell and they were desperate.

It's hard to do a thorough rectal examination in a 10-month old kitten, but there seemed to be no anal or rectal obstruction. Radiographs

---

4 Bernarde A, Viguier E. Transpelvic urethrostomy in 11 cats using an ischial ostectomy. *Veterinary Surgery* 2004; 33: 246–252.

did not show a foreign body. Her pelvic diameter was not compromised and her caudal neurologic function was normal. My surgical colleague, who was the primary clinician on this case, agreed that Alicja might benefit from a colectomy and she was scheduled for surgery. Curious about the condition of megacolon in general, I watched them do it.

When her abdomen was opened, Alicja's colon bulged out like a huge Kielbasa sausage. Outwardly, it resembled megacolon, except that rather than being filled with dehydrated fecoliths, it was distended with a gritty paste liberally seasoned with psyllium and grated ginger. It was much more compatible with chronic partial obstruction. As the surgeon explored Alicja's caudal abdomen, it became evident that her colon was being occluded by an extraluminal band of fibrous tissue. Sclerosing adenocarcinoma can have a similar appearance, but she would have to be the unluckiest kitten in the world. Similarly, segmental colonic obstruction can occur with feline infectious peritonitis. But this obstruction was very focal, and did not seem associated with any mass. It was as if a band of elastic tissue had encircled the colorectal junction and was tethering it to the …

"Uterine body!" exclaimed the surgical student.

Indeed, on further examination, the cause of Alicja's obstruction became apparent. When Alicja was spayed, her two uterine horns had been tied together – midway down – within a single ligature. The remnants of her two uterine horns and her uterine body were encircling her colon and causing extraluminal compression, rather like a vascular ring anomaly. Coincidentally, this surgical complication had first been reported by another colleague of mine, Peter Muir.[5]

The only way you could physically achieve this result would be to pull one uterine horn up the side of the colon, and the other horn *through*

a defect in the mesocolon, then place a clamp across both of them. I could imagine a scenario where the spay hook pushed through the mesentery dorsal to the colon; after which the uterine horns were exteriorized and ligated with minimal visualization. This time and suture-saving measure, however, had cost Alicja and her owners dearly.

The good news was that Alicja had a treatable problem, and maybe her colon could recover if the obstruction was relieved. The uterine ring anomaly was released by transecting one uterine horn, dissecting the remnants from the colonic serosa, and completing her spay by ligating the uterus just above the cervix. Almost immediately, the colon in that region began to dilate as fecal mush pushed past it. We could only hope that the colonic muscle would regain normal peristalsis. We knew that cats with colonic obstruction secondary to pelvic fractures, for instance, did not always regain the ability to defecate normally even when their orthopedic issues were corrected.

Alicja beat the odds, however, and recovered completely. She was not my patient, but she remains one of the most memorable.

Bluey is another. He was eight years old when he began straining. Like Alicja, he failed medical management for his megacolon, but in his case abdominal sonography revealed a cavitated mass in his pelvic inlet. Had he been a dog, rather than a Bengal, we would have diagnosed a prostatic cyst, but, being a cat, surely that was unlikely?

It proved to be the precise cause of his problem. The radiologists aspirated purulent material and we treated Bluey just like a dog with a prostatic abscess. Being a cat, he had more than enough omentum for the job, and decompressing his cavitated prostate cured his constipation – temporarily at least. But the pus proved sterile, and the biopsy revealed an underlying prostatic adenocarcinoma, and Bluey sadly did not live very long.

Jemima had a happier outcome, although things looked shaky for a while. She, too, presented for

---

5 Muir P, Goldsmid SE, Bellenger CR. Megacolon in a cat following ovariohysterectomy. *Veterinary Record* 1991; 129: 512–513.

chronic straining and a perineal mass. The perineal mass proved to be a large fecal accumulation that recurred repeatedly after removal under anesthesia, and intermittently "calved" tenacious dollops of excreta onto her family's bespoke rugs. Dietary manipulation failed to cure the problem and although Jemima's colon was not as distended as other cats we had seen, some variant of megacolon seemed the most likely explanation.

I wasn't convinced. Had Jemima been a dog, we would have been highly suspicious of perineal hernia. But she was a Persian cat, and she did not have a classic perineal hernia; there was no soft tissue bulge, no eccentric sacculation of the rectum. It seemed, though, that her problem was focused in the perineum and rectum, not the colon.

I told the owners, "I need to palpate her under anesthesia."

Palpation ruled out a true perineal hernia. However, there was very little strength to Jemima's perineal diaphragm. I could hook the tip of my little finger laterally from her rectum and see it bulging through the skin beside the anus.

"I think she has perineal laxity," I told the resident and student. "It's not a classic perineal *hernia*, but the muscles of the perineal diaphragm are weak and can't exert sufficient lateral force on the rectum during defecation." I exhausted my technical vocabulary at that point, "So the feces just squishes around cranial to the anus, rather than coming out."

We see the same thing in dogs, particularly on the contralateral side to a classic perineal hernia. I suspect it is the reason problems recur in some patients. Neither side is normal, but we only repair the side that has failed to the point of visceral herniation. The weak side then gets more and more lax until it also herniates. We call all defects of the perineal diaphragm perineal *hernias*, but it might be more helpful to describe the muscle weakness as perineal *laxity*, instead. If the patient is showing signs of difficult defecation, though, surgical repair seems indicated regardless of whether or not a discrete defect (hernial ring) has opened in the pelvic canal.

Jemima was a great illustration of this dilemma. I recommended herniorrhaphy to treat her suspected perineal laxity, but I was nervous because I didn't know for sure that it was the cause of her signs. It wasn't described in the literature, but it made so much sense.

As much as they loved her, Jemima's parents were growing tired of cleaning their rugs, and felt she was becoming – not only physically distressed – but also exceedingly embarrassed by these events. They decided to take the risk.

Two days after surgery, Jemima walked to her litter box, squatted, and passed a column of feces that would have done a German Shepherd proud. Her look of relief was probably only surpassed by mine.

If you are going to tackle perineal herniorrhaphy in a cat – or in a young puppy – expect muscle bellies like strips of raw chicken breast. They can be hard to differentiate from subcutaneous fat, and if you are in any way visually challenged, wear glasses or operating loupes. Don't use thick suture material; your challenge is to coax these flimsy tissues together, rather than forcing them. And clip right past the greater trochanter to give you scope to reinforce the repair with a superficial gluteal muscle flap. These cases probably should be performed in a perineal stand (rather than ventral recumbency; see Chapter 10), in order to access the superficial gluteal if you need it.

The moral of these seemingly disconnected stories? Distended colons aren't all *megacolons*. There are lots of reasons for colonic distention in cats and if I have encountered so many, you will too.

It seemed we were having a run on megacolon cases, and one of our surgery residents, Penny Tisdall, was researching the myenteric plexus in affected cats, when Bandit came to see us.

Bandit broke the mold; although the size of your average cat, and living a cat-like lifestyle in an inner-city apartment, he had been born a dog. Nevertheless, he was having trouble defecating, and his colon was permanently distended despite being fed chicken and rice, laced with increasing volumes of lactulose. Bandit's problems started with a single episode of constipation from which he never recovered.

"It's unusual for a dog to have megacolon," I told the referring vet. "And all the surgeons I've asked say they avoid colectomy in the dog like the plague. I think he has a horrible prognosis if we go there."

"Can you look at him for me and tell that to his owners? They don't want to hear it from me."

"No worries."

Bandit was a cute Maltese with blackcurrant eyes and a cotton boll face. He was friendly, despite his humans' unnatural fascination with his back end. But his bouncing play was punctuated by frequent episodes of squatting and straining, to no apparent end.

He was an enigma. His colon was distended with feces, but it was soft. I could pass a finger through his anus and – with patience – right into his terminal colon. He had good anal tone and a loud yelp suggested normal sensation. I found no good reason why he couldn't defecate. I suggested my resident also examine him.

"I can't get my finger in," she said after a few moments.

"Really? I got in just fine."

"Nope, I can feel some sort of ledge …" she swiveled her hand around. "Ah, there it goes." Her finger slid in to the second knuckle. "Weird."

I began to palpate him again, but by now we were stretching the friendship to its breaking point, and Bandit called time-out on this increasingly unpleasant game.

We returned the next day with Bandit asleep and relaxed. I found little resistance to passing my finger as long as I angled it craniodorsally. But if I tried advancing in a cranioventral direction, I hit a tight band on the floor of the rectum, which caused the tissues to buckle like a flap-valve. Once beyond the shelf, however, I squished into a morass of fecal putty.

I placed a vaginal speculum to view Bandit's terminal rectum. There was a distinct fibrous band across the ventral third, about a centimeter cranial to the anus.

"Is it a stricture?" someone asked. Perhaps it was me, because no-one answered.

"I think it's a stricture," I said, more definitively.

"Can we balloon it?"

I think we could have ballooned it, but it was so close to the anus …

"Perhaps we can just incise it," I said.

"Won't it just constrict down again?"

"Not if I incise it longitudinally, and then–" *assiduous epithelial to epithelial apposition* – "perhaps I can suture the wound transversely."

Breathing a thank you to Heineke and Miculicz – those creative Polish surgeons – I flushed the rectum with chlorhexidine, grasped a No. 11 blade and performed a simple "rectoplasty." It took all of five minutes. I sutured the partial-thickness longitudinal defect transversely, which opened the rectum to the extent that I could have passed my thumb up there had I felt the need. Not wanting to jinx things, I restricted the resident and student to little fingers, as they all wanted to confirm elimination of the valve effect.

I went to tell Bandit's owners the news.

"Fingers crossed until we see whether this helps," I warned them.

Three hours later, we walked a slightly ataxic Bandit onto the lawn outside the horse yard. Based on previous experience, we expected him to trot around for a while, presumably preparing himself for the inevitable disappointment when he did finally squat. We were so sure he would do this that we almost missed it when he strained and a huge coil of feces burst from his anus. Due to his diet of chicken and rice, it bore a disturbing resemblance to toothpaste leaving a tube. After that, there was more, and then a little more. Shocked, Bandit spun around to investigate this colossal deposit. When I palpated his abdomen, his colon was empty.

We later learned that Bandit received an enema during his first episode of constipation. I will never know whether he had a stricture then or not. Was the mucosal damage that led to the stricture caused by a foreign body that passed without anyone seeing it, or a rigid enema nozzle?

It didn't matter. I was just happy I didn't have to remove Bandit's colon in order to make him poop again. It would be several more years before I was forced to do that to a dog.[6]

---

6 Sarathchandra SK, Lunn JA, Hunt GB. Ligation of the caudal mesenteric artery during resection and anastomosis of the colorectal junction for annular adenocarcinoma in two dogs. *Australian Veterinary Journal* 2009; 87: 356–359.

18

"An Alien in My Waiting Room"

Everyday Occurences of the Unexpected and Unbelievable

I saw so many cases with pelvic canal obstruction resulting from masses at the pelvic inlet that I was confident, when they contacted me about Charlie, we would get to the bottom of his problem – so to speak.

Charlie was straining to defecate and urinate. He was a very unhappy boy, and in the last five days had eaten a single – peeled – grape, which might have been an odd dietary choice, had Charlie not been a golden lion tamarin. Charlie weighed 600 g, but that didn't change our approach. Ultrasonography showed an amorphous mass right at his pelvic inlet and an FNA yielded little except red blood cells and fibrin. It clearly wasn't an abscess, but what was it?

Having experienced success with similar patients suffering from necrotic lipomas, fibromas, leiomyomas, and paraprostatic cysts, I suggested the best option was surgical exploration. Charlie's size didn't worry me; if we could reduce an intussusception in a leopard gecko, ligate a patent ductus arteriosus in a 700-g kitten, and remove an ovarian cyst from a goldfish, Charlie should be well within our limits. I had learned the necessity of having a set of petite instruments, surgical magnification, and good lighting. I had also learned, courtesy of a troublesome guinea pig, that the tissues in these tiny patients are very fragile, so Q-tips (cotton buds) are a must. But they also dry out easily, so moistening the Q-tips with saline is also mandatory. I ran through the procedure with the exotics resident and Faculty; we would perform a standard ventral midline laparotomy (a luxury we did

not have in reptiles, for instance, because of their superficial ventral vein).

I had done little surgery on primates. They usually came from zoos and research facilities, and when their own highly experienced vets needed help they called in human surgeons. I had participated in a lung biopsy in an orangutan many years before, assisting one of Sydney's best-known human cardiothoracic surgeons, but am not sure what help I really offered, captivated as I was by our patient's massive hands and indescribable smell.

I wondered how I would feel, operating on one of my simian cousins. Once the drapes are on, though, tissues are tissues and anatomy is anatomy, and tackling Charlie's abdomen was little different to that of a chinchilla or a rabbit (or anything furry in which the internal anatomy is unfamiliar). Some gentle redistribution of viscera, probing with a moist Q-tip, and I had isolated the firm, round mass occluding Charlie's pelvic inlet. It was minimally vascular and covered in a grayish capsule. It didn't have a pulse, and when I aspirated it again with a 25-gauge needle, it did not bleed. The small rent in the outer fibrous layer gaped slightly to expose something dark and firm that looked remarkably like an organizing blood clot. It didn't seem attached to the viscera, and although I could not see the terminal branches of the aorta, the ultrasound and our aspirations suggested it wasn't vascular. Was it an old hemorrhage in the lymph node? Or maybe a paraprostatic cyst? I had seen necrotic lipomas in this region that looked similar. We didn't know *what* it was, but it needed to

Pitfalls in Veterinary Surgery, First Edition. Edited by Geraldine B. Hunt.
© 2017 John Wiley & Sons, Inc. Published 2017 by John Wiley & Sons, Inc.

come out, or we should probably euthanize Charlie on the table, as he was miserable and in pain. So I incised slowly through the fibrous capsule.

Nothing bad happened. The capsule peeled back to reveal a rubbery black nodule that shelled out with minimal manipulation. Had I known it to be neoplastic, I would have been more circumspect about Charlie's prognosis, but it seemed simply to be a blood clot, and if I could remove it, Charlie's symptoms should resolve.

As a surgeon, though, I always want to go one step further. I had removed the major portion of the presumed blood clot but I wasn't satisfied. I wanted the last little fragment so I advanced my Q-tip into the depths of the capsule.

A pool of blood welled in Charlie's abdomen. There was no asking the student, "Can you work out how much blood Charlie has?" or "How much does he have to lose before it becomes clinically relevant?" I just stuck my finger in the hole. Fortunately, Charlie's abdomen was so small, and my finger so large, that there was little room for anything else.

Forget about bleeding you can *hear*. I had been trained to think that in our tiny exotic patients, the carnival was over if you encountered bleeding you could even *see*. I must have torn something with that last rub of the Q-tip.

Darn!

Now what? As far as the anesthetist was concerned, Charlie still seemed to be stable. But if I removed my finger to see what was going on, that was likely to change in a hurry.

Use first principles. I told myself. *This is a tiny patient, and an unusual species, but his blood should still clot.*

I suctioned the pooled blood from around my finger (thankfully, no more appeared) and waited, for at least five minutes, while goodness-knew-whatever rent in Charlie's great pelvic vessels sealed itself. During that time, I made plans. I had the operating room tech open some Gelfoam™ onto the surgery tray. My student cut it into 1-cm squares, ready to pack into the defect once I summoned the courage to remove my finger.

This is good enough for battlefield surgeons, I told myself, *so it should be good enough for Charlie.*

Except … was it?

"This is it," I told the student, resident, and anesthetist – and the crowd of onlookers that grew as news of this horribly fascinating development spread.

I grasped a wad of Gelfoam in forceps with my left hand, and slowly withdrew my finger from Charlie's abdomen. The bloody tide did not rise immediately, so I jammed the Gelfoam into the defect, and placed a surgical sponge on top of that.

"So far so good."

We lavaged the abdomen gently, tidied our table, and got everything we needed for closure. If Charlie's bleeding stopped, I thought, it would be a miracle.

"Don't lose that blood clot," I warned the student. "We need to submit it for histopath. And," – half wishing I hadn't removed it in the first place – "we definitely *don't* want it going back in the patient!"

Charlie did not bleed any more, and I palpated his now-patent pelvic inlet before I closed his abdomen.

Despite coming so close to meeting his tamarin maker, Charlie recovered slowly but completely, and began to pass urine and feces again within hours of surgery. Having developed a taste for peeled grapes, he chose them above other offerings for the next few days, but everyone agreed that he was doing well.

My phone rang late the following week. Being very diligent, Charlie's doctors had decided to perform a follow-up abdominal ultrasound. They were disturbed to see a mass of similar texture and in exactly the same location as the original blood clot. Coagulated Gelfoam, it turns out, looks remarkably similar to clots of other types.

"How is he doing?" I asked.

"He's great. He seems back to normal."

"And … ?" *What are you asking me, exactly?*

"I don't think we want to go back in, do we?"

They didn't make me tell them that if they wanted the Gelfoam removed they were going to have to do it themselves!

"Gelfoam is supposed to be absorbable. Hopefully it will shrink."

"Yes. Hopefully."

I related this story late one evening at an American College of Veterinary Surgeons meeting. There was some beer involved and we were trading weird surgical cases.

"So I removed the clot," I said, "and it … "

"… bled?"

"Yes!"

"Well, what did you expect? I mean, a blood clot is usually there for a reason."

I had expected a little more compassion, but then, we *were* a bunch of surgeons.

"Well …" I didn't have a good answer. I suppose the fact that I didn't know why the blood clot had occurred in the first place made me feel the bleeding might not happen again.

"I mean … *duh!*"

Fortunately, I liked this particular surgeon and thus was able to control the urge to pour my beer over his head.

But it did make me wonder what the blood clot was all about. Despite my medical and surgical knowledge, though, it took an article in that august journal, *The Hollywood Reporter*, to ignite the flame of an idea, and an old friend's medical emergency to fan it.

Two things happened in the same week: Sharon Stone opened up to Merle Ginsberg about her cerebral aneurysm[1] and – half a world away – an 80-year-old ocean swimmer suffered excruciating pain in his right leg. Both people ended up with stents as a result of arterial aneurysms.

The Greeks called this type of development *deus ex machina*, whereby a "seemingly unsolvable problem is suddenly and abruptly resolved by the inspired and unexpected intervention of some new event, character, ability or object."[2]

I call it luck.

Could Charlie have had a thrombosed iliac aneurysm? It made me cold to think that I had blithely opened it and scooped out the clot. It might make sense, though. I had been thinking about diseases of dogs and cats, whereas I should have been thinking about those of primates. A literature search revealed that tamarins do, indeed, develop aortic aneurysms, although they are usually closer to the heart.[3] I don't know whether that was the reason for Charlie's clot, but it could certainly explain the torrential bleeding when I teased it away. On an afternoon when I had nothing better to do, curiosity took me to the human literature, where I learned that an unfortunate Canadian gentleman had clinical signs very similar to Charlie's caused by a thrombosed iliac aneurysm.[4]

Sometimes, despite all the knowledge and equipment at our disposal, we still have to fly by the seat of our pants.

Would I have treated Charlie any differently had I suspected an aneurysm? Almost certainly. I would have been far more pessimistic, for a start. Gelfoam isn't a *bad* thing to treat an aneurysm, it's just that most people would apply it through a catheter, rather than an arteriotomy. That would have been a sweet challenge for our interventionalists and I feel a little guilty for depriving them of it.

I was happy, though, that despite completely overlooking this common primate disease, following the basic principles of surgery had carried me and Charlie to a satisfactory outcome.

---

1 Sharon Stone opens up about about her brain aneurysm: "I spent two years learning to walk and talk again." *Hollywood Reporter* 2014. http://www.hollywoodreporter.com/news/sharon-stone-opens-up-her-755488

2 Wikipedia.

3 Gozalo AS, Ragland DR, StClaire MC, Elkins WR, Michaud CR. Intracardiac thrombosis and aortic dissecting aneurysms in mustached tamarins (*Saguinus mystax*) with cardiomyopathy. *Comparative Medicine* 2011; 61(2): 176–181.

4 Elkouri S, Blair J, Beaudoin N, Bruneau L. Ruptured solitary internal iliac artery aneurysm: a rare cause of large-bowel obstruction. *Canadian Journal of Surgery* 2008; 51(6): E122–E123.

Sometimes the "alien in your waiting room" is not your patient, but its disease.

Even with well-heeled owners who wanted the very best, Fanta was always going to be a challenge. The previously gentle, middle-aged Labrador cross presented with one eye partially closed, foul-smelling fluid dripping from sinus tracts around her eye and ear, and an intermittent nasal discharge (Figure 18.1A). She was exquisitely head-shy, resented anyone coming near her, and screamed when she opened her mouth to bite them. Needless to say, she was one bad prognosis away from euthanasia.

"She's always been so healthy," her owner sniffled through a wet handkerchief. "Then she started scratching her ear … and now *this*." Her sniffles became sobs. "She won't even let us pet her any more!"

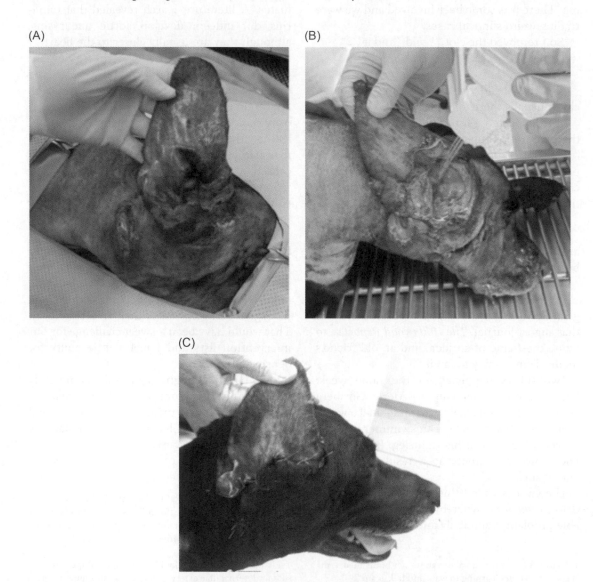

(A)

(B)

(C)

Figure 18.1 (A) Extensive draining sinuses in a dog with chronic otitis externa and media. (B) Treatment of an open wound following total ear canal ablation. (C) Local healing complete after secondary wound closure.

"It's time," her husband said quietly.

Looking at Fanta, I found it hard to disagree.

"Whatever she has, even if it's treatable ... it's so far advanced," I said. Although the ubiquitous foxtail had been mentioned in the referral letter, my gut was telling me that rampant adenocarcinoma, or some deep-seated fungal infection was more likely.

"I know, I know. I don't want to put her through any more. But I have to *know* ..." she interrupted herself with sobs, "that there's nothing we can do."

How could we know what was needed unless we knew what we were treating? I searched the surgical textbook for the chapter *"Fetid oozing sinuses on dog's face"* to no avail, so I was going to have to work from first principles.

We agreed on examination under anesthesia, otoscopy, FNA, CT, and deep tissue culture. Although Fanta would not feel anything during this process, I didn't like the thought of committing her owners to all that expense if her prognosis was horrible.

"Let's take it step by step," I suggested. "If at any time we find something we know we can't fix – we'll stop and make a decision." I didn't think we would get very far.

Examination of her caudal oral cavity was unremarkable. Otoscopy showed some otitis externa, and a pus-rimmed hole where her eardrum should be, but nothing exceptionally bad. No foxtails, unfortunately. Repeated FNAs showed inflammatory cells and bacteria, but despite heroic efforts on our part and that of the cytologist, absolutely no indication of neoplasia. Contrast-enhanced CT was the kicker. I was expecting some advanced, osteolytic process eating away at the tympanic bulla, maybe even the temporomandibular joint. What I saw was disease focused entirely on the tympanic bulla, the ossified ear canal of chronic otitis externa, a mess of soft tissue inflammation and fibrosis, and myriad draining sinuses extending to the orbit, the parotid region, and into the nasopharynx. No fungi were evident microscopically, although Fanta had acquired a collection of bacteria worthy of an award.

"The ear seems to be the main source of the problem," I told her owners, who were sitting in the waiting room. As so often happens, in chatting with the other clients in the waiting room, they had started an informal otitis support group, and the Masons were telling them what a miracle Moose's ear canal ablation had proved to be.

"Can you remove it?"

"I can remove the ear canal, and clean out the middle ear. But I can't remove all the infected tissue, it's extending too far."

"But if you treat the infection ..."

"It may be hard to treat the infection if we can't remove all the abnormal tissue that's causing it in the first place."

I knew there was a reasonable risk of chronic infection and refractory draining sinus even in the best of cases, and Fanta was hardly that. I could envision removing Fanta's ear canal, but the prospect of closing the oozing wound was unpalatable. And then there was the issue of which antibiotic to use.

"We'll leave the wound open," I decided out loud. "It means we will have to go back and close it in a few days, once the tissues start looking healthier" – *if the tissues start looking healthier.*

"You mean treat it as an open wound?" the student asked when we discussed it later in rounds. We treated a lot of *open* wounds as open wounds, but we weren't in the habit of simply leaving surgical sites open. At least, not when they involved a named structure like the *tympanic bulla.*

"Yep."

It will be interesting to see if that works. Even I was wondering.

I had to chisel Fanta's mineralized ear canal from the base of her skull, and rongeur her bulla loudly enough that I was sure she would react despite the pharmacologic cocktail keeping her asleep. I told her owners that she would not blink again; her facial nerve was surely enveloped in mineralized and infected tissue. Having removed the ear canal, and carved a generous slot in the lateral aspect of her bulla, I began probing the sinus tracts. All roads lead to Rome, and in this case, all sinus tracts led to a point at the membranous junction with her osteum, where the infection had grown bored with the external ear canal, found a weak spot, and gone walkabout through the complex structures of her retropharynx.

"Do you have to open them all up?"

I ran a red rubber tube into each sinus and flushed it vigorously. "I don't think so. They don't have an epithelial lining, so assuming we have removed the main focus, and they continue to drain effectively, they should heal up." *Should.*

The large hole I had created in the side of Fanta's head now looked remarkably healthy. I packed it with a silver-impregnated polyure-thane foam dressing and tied over two laparot-omy pads, which obviated the need for a bandage around Fanta's head. We applied drops to protect her eye, as she would not be able to protect it herself, and wheeled her into post-anesthetic recovery. I still felt ambivalent about her prognosis, but at least I knew the pus that would almost certainly accumulate under her bandage had an easy way to the surface, and no longer needed to track out through her orbit, or her nasopharynx.

Four days later, we anesthetized Fanta for the last time, lavaged her granulating wound, and sutured it over a closed-suction drain (Figure 18.1B). Even better, the microbial sus-ceptibility report returned a remarkably benign profile, so we prescribed amoxicillin-clavulanic acid for the foreseeable future.

Ten days later, Fanta returned for suture and drain removal. She was a completely different dog; she was back to her affectionate and happy self. Her right eye, previously bloodshot and blinking away rancid pus, was clear and open and – blinking! Her draining sinuses were no more than discolored dimples, and her surgical wound was completely healed. Somebody was looking out for her (Figure 18.1C).

Two months later, I used the same technique on an almost identical case. The confounding variable was that, after agreeing to the compre-hensive work-up including CT, Choc Top's owner announced that she had no more money

for treatment, and certainly could *not* afford a week in hospital with open wound manage-ment, followed by a *second* surgical procedure to close the wound. No *way*, no *how*!

"You sucked me into agreeing to this," she said, "and now you're taking advantage of me."

In some small measure, I agreed with her. Although we had been professional and thor-ough, we might have done a better job of walk-ing her through the likely costs for treatment once we had identified the cause of the problem. In defense of the consulting doctor, open wound management followed by delayed closure attracts a significant charge. And it wasn't our fault that our culture yielded a methicillin-resistant staphylococcus with all its attendant complications.

"So I am going to have to put him to sleep, *and* I have this big bill – all for nothing!"

So, who you gonna call when this sort of excreta strikes the ventilation system and you have a packed schedule of consults and cases breathing down your neck?

"I really want to work something out," I told our client services manager, who had agreed to take over communications while my resident and I attended to other patients. "I think we can help Choc Top, and maybe it doesn't have to cost an arm and a leg."

Choc Top was a rotund, black and white, Fox Terrier style of dog. I hadn't met his owner, but I knew she drove big rigs for a living. Our conver-sations had taken place via tenuous telephone connections on which we competed with static as she trucked from one state to another, which was at least partly responsible for the impasse at which we had now arrived.

"She has a strict financial limit. And she can't afford the fancy antibiotics you are suggesting." These weren't the client services manager's words, she was quoting Choc Top's owner. Had I felt less responsible for the situation, I might have taken offense, or at least tried to explain our reasons, but that wasn't going to help. So I swallowed my ego and focused on the end game, which was getting Choc Top's ear canal out in the hope that his body could take care of the rest.

"How about we cap the cost for the ear canal ablation? She takes the dog home the day after surgery and does her own dressing changes."

"She says she can manage that. But she can't afford to come back for wound closure."

"Then let's not close the wound," I said. "It can heal by second intention." It was only a small advance on what we did with Fanta. There was barely any tension on the wound following an ear canal ablation. I had seen massive abscess cavities on the side of the neck heal, so why not this one?

"If we leave the wound open we might be able to get away with topical treatment. But she would have to keep an eye out for any signs that Choc Top is getting sick from a deep infection that isn't resolving, in which case he really needs the 'fancy' antibiotics."

"Yes, she understands that."

We had a compromise plan. Did I feel good sending a patient home with an open wound and no plans to close it? Perhaps I should have, but I would have felt worse euthanizing Choc Top, otherwise someone would have had to cover the cost of hospitalization, barrier nursing, and wound reconstruction.

You couldn't do it with every client; there must be a selection process; but in this case, Choc Top's owner did everything that was required. She created her own absorbent bandages with sanitary pads and stockinette, applied honey and then Silvazine – all of which she could buy at the local shopping center – and let nature take its course. Unwilling to return Choc Top for fear of incurring more expense, she kept in touch with our client services manager. I was told that Choc Top's wound healed within two weeks.

Sometimes the "alien in your waiting room" is not your patient, or it's disease, but your client.

Bree's Mom was completely unreadable. While her husband was chatty and nodded when I was speaking to acknowledge that – even if he didn't understand or particular like what I was saying – at least I was saying something.

Bree's Mom sat stony faced, did not speak, and barely moved. Her only expression was a faint scowl that suggested I was the root cause

of all their problems and if I would simply cease breathing they could all relax and return to their normal lives. I like to think I can connect quickly with people, in fact I *need* that reassurance in order to feel comfortable taking a case on. Bree had a serious problem that required complex surgery and I needed to know that her owners trusted me and were listening. I got absolutely nothing from Mrs. Rosetta Lapidus. Putting aside my first impression – that she hated me – I worked through some alternatives. Was English a problem for her? I doubted it. Was she simply trying to concentrate on what I was saying? Possible. I have known colleagues who frown and stare unnervingly when I am speaking; not because they disagree, but because they want to make sure they understand. I suspect I do it myself.

Rosetta quite probably mistrusted me, which might have nothing to do with me or my reputation, and everything to do with her personality and the time it might take her to open up to a new person.

Or was she scared? I recalled the seemingly hostile stares of generations of veterinary students when I corrected the way they were holding their instruments in a practical exam, and how I eventually recognized them as the mute manifestation of terror.

Yes, fear was a distinct possibility, given the circumstances.

Whatever the explanation, I needed to sort it out before we could engage in a meaningful discussion of Bree's illness and – hopefully – make some good decisions.

What is Rosetta's button? I asked myself. *Where is the dial I can use to tune into her wavelength?*

Being highly trained professionals, it is tempting to fall back on our knowledge, our experience, and our qualifications. If only we can show these people how competent we are, surely they will trust us? Or perhaps not. They might *tolerate* us, they might *agree* with us, they might *pay* us, but trust is much harder to come by.

Let's say Rosetta was as suspicious and hostile as she appeared – which was not necessarily deliberate as she might not have a clue how she projected – but let's say she *was*. What would I need to do, to break through that wall?

In teaching students, I feel they respect me more if they understand me. They seem more likely to engage when they see me as human; at least somewhat like them. I feel I am a better role model when I can show them I have interests, passions, loves, and fears.

Would this approach work with Rosetta? I doubted it. Although it is a good way to connect with some people, many clients are not that simple. What I had to learn by experience – and I am sure people far more knowledgeable than I have written and lectured on the topic – is that vets and our clients share one important common interest. Their animal; be it pet, companion, employee, or carer.

Rosetta was not here because of *me*. She was here because of Bree.

Bree would be the button.

I kneeled on the floor and let the dog come to me.

"I love Gordon Setters," I said. "I used to own one." I ran my hand along her side. "She feels so soft. Are you naturally soft?" I asked the dog. "Or do your humans brush you?"

"She's naturally soft." Three words from Rosetta. Awesome!

I caught her eye. "I'm sorry Bree has this problem. I want you to know that my goal is to work out what is best for her. Not what is possible, or what might work for another dog, but what works for *her*."

Rosetta nodded. "That's what we want."

"I can give you my professional opinion," I said. "But first, tell me what *you* want for Bree?"

And suddenly, the stone Rosetta was gone: her face animated and she began to talk. "I don't want her to suffer after surgery …"

"Well fortunately we can control that with medication …"

Which was good, because Bree's surgery was complicated, and her recovery was even more complicated, and every time we spoke to the Lapidi we had to increase her estimate and downgrade her prognosis. Eventually, we had to transfer her to the intensivists – never a good outcome when your patient enters the hospital with vital organs in perfect working order – regardless of their skill! But they worked their magic, the beeping machines did their job, and Bree did hers, and she went home almost a month later.

By which time Rosetta not only smiled occasionally, but was on hugging terms with everyone.

The final species of "alien" that we encounter from time to time is not human or animal, or even vegetable or mineral. It comes from nowhere, it is intangible and it is very, very hard to explain. It is the "gut feeling."

Moreton's owner was made up something serious. Black eyeliner, lashes laquered to the point of rigidity, rouged cheeks, cherry-red lips that went perfectly with Moreton's painted toenails, and her scarf a vivid match to the scrunchie restraining his top-knot.

"It's the noise. I can hear it from the other side of the room!" she said.

Moreton was seated in the corner of the consulting room, examining his private parts. Hard as I might try, I could hear nothing other than the sound of licking.

"A squeaking noise, can't you hear it?"

Whether I could hear it or not was immaterial. The noise had prompted Jonique to take Moreton to her vet, who shortly thereafter auscultated a high-pitched ejection-type murmur emanating from his right heart base.

"That's new," she said, having examined Moreton only three months previously for his annual wellness check.

The cardiologists identified a mass attached to his pulmonic valve, popping in and out of view like a ball valve (Figure 18.2A).

I talked Jonique through the mechanics and risks of total venous inflow occlusion under hypothermia. Considering that Moreton was currently healthy, I gave my chances of tackling this fascinating surgery as close to zero.

"What are his chances of survival?"

I gave Jonique her the magical – and arbitrary – number, "Fifty percent."

(A)

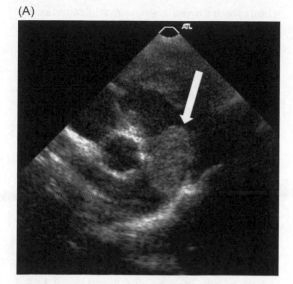

(B)

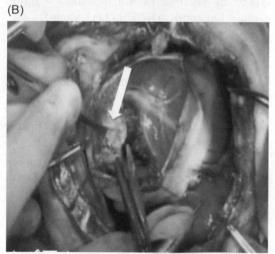

Figure 18.2 (A) Echocardiogram showing myxoma (arrow) of the pulmonic valve annulus causing a loud ejection-type murmur in a dog. (B) This tumor (arrow) was removed successfully through a ventriculotomy of the right ventricular outflow tract under total venous inflow occlusion.

She fixed me with painted eyes. "My daughter is an entertainer. When she was 18, she wanted to move to New York to get into the dancing scene. I said, *You go for it, girl.*"

Not the advice most of my friends would have given their children.

"Now she is in a musical on Broadway."

Not the outcome I was expecting, either.

"I have a good feeling about this surgery," said Jonique. "I heard the tumor talking to me. I have no doubt that's what happened, and that's why we caught it when we did. Well, Moreton is telling me he has a good feeling, too. So, as I said to my daughter, *You go for it, girl!*"

I held that thought as I clamped Moreton's cranial and caudal vena cava, and his azygous vein, and watched his heart empty of blood. I held it as I palpated the firm lump of his pulmonic tumor. I held it as I incised the pulmonary outflow tract and teased the mass from its attachment to the valve annulus (Figure 18.2B). I vented air from his heart and closed the incision with a continuous polypropylene suture, and then I held my breath until it started pumping effectively again.

"I never doubted it!" said Jonique when I told her Moreton was breathing on his own in ICU.

In Moreton's case, his owner's positive thinking paid off.

More often it goes the other way; so much so that I have learned never to ignore gut feelings, be they mine or my clients'.

"If you have a bad feeling about this," I say, "perhaps we shouldn't go ahead."

If something goes wrong, or even right, it will be the gut feeling we remember. Not the test results, the radiology report, or the surgical consent form. If we had a bad feeling, and things go bad, we will wish we had listened to our inner self.

Sometimes, it seems, our gut knows things that we do not.

The thing all these cases have in common is that, despite years of experience, I had to work through them from first principles; using my experience with the known to solve the unknown puzzle. The "aliens" in your waiting room may be different, and they may become progressively more complicated through the years, but they will all be equally exotic and enigmatic until you decode them by using your wits and intuition. Perhaps this also speaks to the "mystery and awe" Dr. Meadows wrote about in Chapter 5.

In my first year as a vet, two perplexing patients came through the door only a week apart.

Rollo was a three-year-old Border Collie; one of those "working dogs" who lives in the farmer's house and plays with the kids. Rollo woke up one day distinctly not himself. He stumbled around the yard, and did not want his breakfast.

When I examined Rollo, he had proprioceptive deficits and leaned against the wall of the consulting room as if he were …

"Drunk," agreed Farmer Tim.

He could have been drunk – like Albert, who lapped the remnant beer from Solo cups lying around after a wild party. Or he might have got into the hash stash – like Blue Boy, the budgerigar – who presented on the floor of his cage, bobbing and stretching his wings in a disturbing impression of John Travolta's *Staying Alive*. Farmer Tim didn't look like he had diversified into illicit agriculture – but in the isolated hills out back of Canberra, who knew?

"Let's do some blood work," I suggested, "and keep Rollo in hospital for observation. I'll give him some intravenous fluids." To which Farmer Tim agreed, for Rollo was a "very valuable" working dog: none of the other dogs mustered the chooks quite so adroitly, and with so little mortality.

I don't recall the exact nature of Rollo's blood test abnormalities, but I suspect they included hypoproteinemia, reduced blood urea nitrogen, elevated alkaline phosphatase, and probably also a low-grade leukocytosis. By the time we fasted Rollo for a day, gave him a shot of antibiotics, and rehydrated him he was back to his normal self.

"But what's wrong with him?" asked Farmer Tim, seeking some tangible dividend from the money he had invested in hematology and biochemistry.

"Some sort of mild liver problem," I would almost certainly have told him.

"What caused it?"

I had no idea. Just as I had no idea what caused the low-grade liver disease in Casper, the Maltese who presented the following week with similar signs. Or in Molly, a six-month-old Shih Tzu who presented for stranguria and from whom we removed a single cystic calculus. Or Patsy, the Australian Cattle Dog, who eventrated five days after I sutured her linea alba with chromic surgical gut when removing *her* cystic calculus – and was euthanized after consuming a large portion of her own jejunum. Or Mia, the Siamese who confounded us with her monthly bouts of torrential hypersialosis.

Or Rambo, the Rottweiler who could barely stagger out to reception the morning after being castrated, causing his owner – recently released from prison on a good behavior bond – to march to the far wall and stand, eyes closed and fists clenched, as he struggled to control his rage and avoid smashing his parole. It was the closest I have ever come to being physically assaulted.

"You've given him something to keep him quiet!" he shouted eventually. "Take a blood sample! I'm going to have it checked out!"

Shaking, I drew blood and handed Rambo's owner the syringe. The blood clotted, and although I suspected he had more than a passing familiarity with drug testing, I doubt he would have known what to do with this sample, but I did what I felt I had to in order to get him out of my waiting room.

I wish I had checked Rambo myself before asking the nurse – a 16-year-old high school student – to discharge him to his owners. I wish I had used a longer-acting suture material in Patsy, and I wish I had analyzed her and Molly's bladder stones.

I had to learn all those lessons the hard way. Hopefully, having read this, you won't.

Looking through the retrospectoscope, I think all these patients most likely had congenital portosystemic shunts (CPS). How ironic, then, that my research career was largely based on this disease whose diagnosis eluded me as a young veterinarian? And even more ironic that my reputation in this area was in large part responsible for the offer of a job at UC Davis and ultimately led to my appointment as a professor of soft tissue surgery. Who would have thought?

I wish I had worked it out in at least one of those early patients!

Figure 18.3 Christmas photo from one of my early portosystemic shunt patients, showing his ambivalence about being dressed as a reindeer.

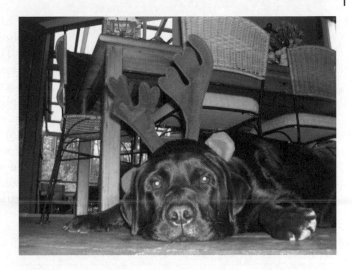

Funnily enough, I have only diagnosed a very few cases of clinically significant congenital portosystemic shunt myself. We picked up some asymptomatic patients during mass screening of breeding dogs for a research paper. Once I became interested in the condition, though, the cases sent to me had already been diagnosed (or the condition strongly suspected) by the referring veterinarian. I merely confirmed what they suspected or ruled it out, or simply went ahead with surgery. That was when the fun started, surely?

But after over 20 years of experience, conducting research, drawing conclusions, developing strategies, leading clients and students through *the spiel* – the benefits of slow occlusion, risk of seizures, portal hypertension, failure to cure, and so on – I discovered that what I knew about CPS in dogs was far outweighed by what I did not.

During the years that my surgical peers and I sought the *best* surgical solution, we merely succeeded in refining a variety of slow occlusion methods that yielded similar results (Figure 18.3). For years, I had been warning owners their dog was less likely to recover if its liver could not return to a normal size. But when my Radiology colleague, Allison Zwingenberger, and I finally studied the change in liver volume using CT angiography, we found

that the dogs who failed to recover – and whose livers failed to grow after surgery – were often those with normal-sized livers in the first place.[5] I had been missing something all those years, and hadn't even known it. Who knows what else I missed?

How would I treat Rollo, were he to present to me tomorrow morning? I would quiz the owners about access to toxins, do a complete physical examination, draw blood for a PCV – at least – and biochemistry. If I found evidence of liver dysfunction (recognizing that cholesterol and blood urea nitrogen can tell you as much about liver function as liver enzymes and bilirubin), I would run pre and postprandial serum bile acids. In the absence of an in-house sonographer, or if the owners were unwilling to pay for one, I would take a lateral abdominal radiograph and evaluate the liver size. And then I might do a treatment trial with a low protein diet, lactulose, and my favorite gastrointestinal antibiotic.

What about CT, scintigraphy, and liver biopsy? All in good time. What point is there,

---

5 Zwingenberger AL, Daniel L, Steffey MA, *et al.* Correlation between liver volume, portal vascular anatomy, and hepatic perfusion in dogs with congenital portosystemic shunt before and after placement of ameroid constrictors. *Veterinary Surgery* 2014; 43(8): 926–934.

unless the owners are prepared to pursue surgical attentuation?

Oh, wait; other types of liver disease occur in young animals and some of those can be treated or at least ameliorated if you can only get a diagnosis.

So how far *should* you go in order to characterize a dog's liver disease? I have no answer to that. But the owners will tell you, once you've clearly outlined their options.

Today, new veterinarians are more likely to diagnose CPS than they are hookworms. Our index of suspicion for this captivating, if not exceptionally common, disease is at an all-time high. The new phase of research into CPS management is focusing on minimally invasive approaches, and better understanding of the pathophysiology in the hope of developing strategies for stimulating liver repair and regeneration. When I graduated, the condition was barely on the radar. What diseases, I wonder, will we see this week that haven't yet been characterized, or whose etiology we still don't understand?

19

Rewind

What Would I Do Differently If I Had the Chance?

In the previous chapters I have described my journey; from veterinary student, to resident, to fully fledged surgeon. I have shared my experiences with soft tissue surgery and hope I have given you an insight as to how I developed an approach to the cases that came through my door, made decisions when the right choice was not obvious, and solved the various puzzles presented to me. Despite the huge amount of information available through lectures and textbooks, there was much I had to learn for myself. Early in my career everything was complicated. As I became more experienced, the common things became routine and I wanted to push the envelope. So I went back to university to forge a career in thoracic and vascular surgery. Cases didn't get much more complex in those days but, as I mastered more and more advanced skills, I started to appreciate the basic cases. I began to enjoy more simple challenges, like trying a different technique, surgical position, or anatomic approach. Studying those experiences in retrospect has brought a clarity that only comes with time and distance.

If I were to pinpoint three key influences that molded me as a clinician, they would be: (i) my early training in anatomy, (ii) the example set by my early mentor, Professor Chris Bellenger, who taught me that surgery is an art form, and (iii) the dogged determination of my close friend and colleague, Richard Malik, with whom I discovered the value of a multidisciplinary approach.

The years have taught me that you cannot pigeonhole diseases by virtue of how they are treated, because the pigeonholes are constantly shuffling. We might think of something as a "surgical disease" or a "medical disease," but that is just a convenient way of categorizing it and maybe making it easier to decide which specialist to refer it to. Send a dog with severe otitis to a surgeon and he loses his ear canal. Send him to a dermatologist and he gets managed medically. Until that doesn't work any longer and *then* he loses his ear canal.

Veterinarians at conferences around the world flock to the spectacle of the *medicine versus surgery* panel discussion, debate, or vigorous disagreement.

Medicine or surgery? Us or them? Which is best?

It seems we focus a lot on *either/or*, whereas the answer is probably somewhere in between. We used to cut the draining tracts from dogs with perianal fistulae; now we treat them with immunosuppressive drugs and only operate on the areas that prove refractory. Similarly with severe otitis externa. Mycobacterial panniculitis used to require massive resection and reconstruction, then we discovered more effective drugs, and now we only reach for the knife when the drugs have failed. These diseases are no longer *surgical*, but they're not completely *medical*, either.

And now, my excellent colleagues from UC Davis, Michele Steffey, Phil Mayhew, and Bill Culp – amongst many others across the

Pitfalls in Veterinary Surgery, First Edition. Edited by Geraldine B. Hunt.
© 2017 John Wiley & Sons, Inc. Published 2017 by John Wiley & Sons, Inc.

world – are showing us that, with the advent of interventional radiology and minimally invasive surgery, even *surgical* diseases are becoming – well – less so. Less invasive is not necessarily less complicated, and certainly isn't less expensive, but few would deny it is far more satisfying.

I can envision a future – maybe not too distant – where lecturers will say, "Can you believe they used to cut animals open? How barbaric was that?"

I have no doubt some of the things I thought I did well – and did routinely – might eventually prove erroneous in the light of future knowledge. Be generous, in years to come, when you look back at the clinical choices you made. You can only work with the information available at the time; your mission is to make the best possible decisions based on that information.

I would love to send this book back in time, so I could read it before starting my own journey (Figure 19.1). If I ever master time travel, I will advise myself to try harder to connect with colleagues and see how they do things, rather than

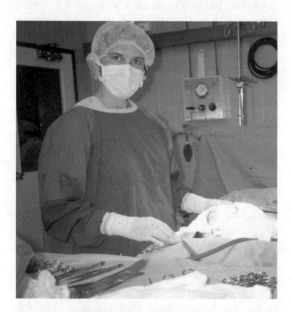

Figure 19.1 Early-career Dr. Hunt looking for inspiration. How much simpler things might have turned out had I been able to read this book back then!

being so focused on my way. I will advise against trying to evaluate cases "on the cheap." Sure, I would work with owners on strategies to limit their costs, but I would try to clarify both in my mind and theirs the compromises required to meet their budget. Admittedly, I am speaking largely from the perspective of a university teaching hospital. But I got caught too many times trying to cut costs by slipping things under the radar; the informal "drive by" ultrasound that is cheap, but scant on information. The brief corridor consultation that sent someone in completely the wrong direction because I failed to follow my own advice and do a thorough physical examination and carefully review all clinical data (including blood test results) in light of what I knew about that patient *on that particular day*.

In a way, cutting costs by strategically picking tests may be more useful to rule things *out* than to rule things *in*. Doing your own cytology (if you're microscopically challenged like me) might serve to prove that something isn't an abscess, but may not provide reliable enough information to make a definitive diagnosis of a soft tissue sarcoma. But that might be alright, if finances are limited and what you really need to know is "Do I have to drain pus?"

I would advise the fledgling "me" to do more ultrasounds. I would get advanced training so I might be able to identify foxtails, as well as abscess cavities, subcutaneous masses, and herniated organs. I would not expect to do full abdominal ultrasounds; a proportion of congenital portosystemic shunts elude even the most experienced sonographers, and if you can't evaluate the pancreas or the dorsocranial abdomen (and try doing that in a patient with a stomach full of food and gas), then you haven't done a thorough job. Couple an amateur ultrasound with a less-than-comprehensive abdominal exploration and you are inviting trouble. Ask the surgeon who removed a mildly distended uterus (mucometra) from a lethargic dog and missed the duodenal linear foreign body because nobody told them to explore the cranial abdomen.

If another surgeon wrote this book, they would have very different experiences to share. No doubt we would have some adventures and misadventures in common, but regardless of how busy our practices are, we really only scratch the surface of our wonderful, complex, intimidating, and vastly rewarding profession. We haven't learned everything there is to know just yet. There is more out there to be discovered, and some of the discoveries will be major; the answers are lurking just below the surface, like Qin Shi Huang's terracotta soldiers. And if a humble farmer can discover the entombed warriors, who says that you might not discover their veterinary equivalent? I hope I have given you courage to exercise your own creativity, to think flexibly, and open your mind to different possibilities and explanations for the perplexing patients you encounter (Figure 19.2).

In sharing my day-by-day challenges I might also have imparted some knowledge that will help you. Perhaps I have given you a head start as you hone your expertise and achieve your own clarity. Maybe I have outlined some strategies for when you really don't know what to do next. At the very least, I hope I provided entertainment and reassurance that you are not the first person to have faced these challenges. Lastly, I would like to think, by describing some

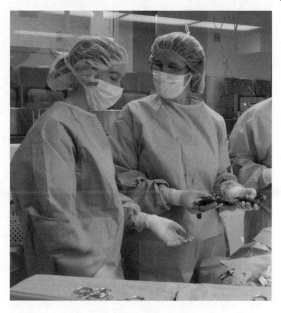

Figure 19.2 Twenty years later, Professor Hunt quizzes a student about the vascular supply to the spleen.

surgical errors and pitfalls, I might protect you from similar mishaps. If this book can save a dog from inadvertent prostatectomy, an owner from wishing he had never signed the consent form, or a veterinarian from doubting she made the right career choice, then it has done its job.

Thank you for reading it.

Index